Physical Healthcare and Promotion in Mental Health Nursing

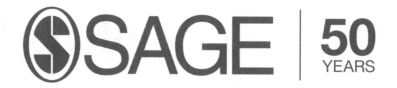

SAGE was founded in 1965 by Sara Miller McCune to support the dissemination of usable knowledge by publishing innovative and high-quality research and teaching content. Today, we publish more than 750 journals, including those of more than 300 learned societies, more than 800 new books per year, and a growing range of library products including archives, data, case studies, reports, conference highlights, and video. SAGE remains majority-owned by our founder, and after Sara's lifetime will become owned by a charitable trust that secures our continued independence.

Los Angeles | London | Washington DC | New Delhi | Singapore

Physical Healthcare and Promotion in Mental Health Nursing

Stan Mutsatsa

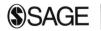

Los Angeles | London | New Delhi
Singapore | Washington DC | Boston

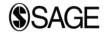

Learning Matters
An imprint of SAGE Publications Ltd
1 Oliver's Yard
55 City Road
London EC1Y 1SP

SAGE Publications Inc.
2455 Teller Road
Thousand Oaks, California 91320

SAGE Publications India Pvt Ltd
B 1/I 1 Mohan Cooperative Industrial Area
Mathura Road
New Delhi 110 044

SAGE Publications Asia-Pacific Pte Ltd
3 Church Street
#10-04 Samsung Hub
Singapore 049483

Editor: Alex Clabburn
Development editor: Caroline Sheldrick
Production controller: Chris Marke
Project management: Swales & Willis Ltd,
Exeter, Devon
Marketing manager: Tamara Navaratnam
Cover design: Wendy Scott
Typeset by: C&M Digitals (P) Ltd, Chennai, India
Printed by: Henry Ling Limited at The Dorset Press,
Dorchester, DT1 1HD

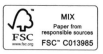

Library of Congress Control Number: 2014958161

British Library Cataloguing in Publication data

A catalogue record for this book is available from the British Library

ISBN 978-1-4462-6817-9
ISBN 978-1-4462-6818-6 (pbk)

At SAGE we take sustainability seriously. Most of our products are printed in the UK using FSC papers and boards. When we print overseas we ensure sustainable papers are used as measured by the Egmont grading system. We undertake an annual audit to monitor our sustainability.

Contents

Transforming Nursing Practice is a series tailor-made for pre-registration student nurses. Each book in the series is:

- ○ Affordable
- ○ Mapped to the NMC Standards and Essential Skills Clusters
- ○ Full of active learning features
- ○ Focused on applying theory to practice

Each book addresses a core topic and they have been carefully developed to be simple to use, quick to read and written in clear language.

"

An invaluable series of books that explicitly relates to the NMC standards. Each book cover a different topic that students need to explore in order to develop into a qualified nurse... I would recommend this series to all Pre-Registration nursing students whatever their field or year of study

Linda Robson
Senior Lecturer, Edge Hill University

The set of books is an excellent resource for students. The series is small, easily portable and valuable. I use the whole set on a regular basis.

Fiona Davies
Senior Nurse Lecturer, University of Derby

I recommend the SAGE/Learning Matters series to all my students as they are relevant and concise. Please keep up the good work.

Thomas Beary
Senior Lecturer in Mental Health Nursing, University of Hertfordshire

"

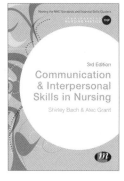

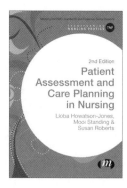

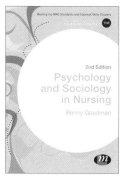

ABOUT THE SERIES EDITORS

Professor Shirley Bach is Head of the School of Health Sciences at the University of Brighton and responsible for the core knowledge titles. Previously she was head of post-graduate studies and has developed curriculum for undergraduate and pre-registration courses in a variety of subject domains.

Dr Mooi Standing is an Independent Academic Consultant (UK and International) and responsible for the personal and professional learning skills titles. She is an accredited NMC Quality Assurance Reviewer of educational programmes and a Professional Regulator Panellist on the NMC Practice Committee.

Sandra Walker is Senior Teaching Fellow in Mental Health at the University of Southampton and responsible for the mental health nursing titles. She is a Qualified Mental Health Nurse with a wide range of clinical experience spanning more than 20 years.

CORE KNOWLEDGE TITLES:

Becoming a Registered Nurse: Making the Transition to Practice
Communication and Interpersonal Skills in Nursing (3rd Ed)
Contexts of Contemporary Nursing (2nd Ed)
Getting into Nursing (2nd Ed)
Health Promotion and Public Health for Nursing Students (2nd Ed)
Introduction to Medicines Management in Nursing
Law and Professional Issues in Nursing (3rd Ed)
Leadership, Management and Team Working in Nursing (2nd Ed)
Learning Skills for Nursing Students
Medicines Management in Children's Nursing
Nursing and Collaborative Practice (2nd Ed)
Nursing and Mental Health Care
Nursing in Partnership with Patients and Carers
Passing Calculations Tests for Nursing Students (3rd Ed)
Palliative and End of Life Care in Nursing
Patient Assessment and Care Planning in Nursing (2nd Ed)
Patient and Carer Participation in Nursing
Patient Safety and Managing Risk in Nursing
Psychology and Sociology in Nursing (2nd Ed)
Successful Practice Learning for Nursing Students (2nd Ed)
Understanding Ethics in Nursing Practice
Using Health Policy in Nursing
What is Nursing? Exploring Theory and Practice (3rd Ed)

PERSONAL AND PROFESSIONAL LEARNING SKILLS TITLES:

Clinical Judgement and Decision Making for Nursing Students (2nd Ed)
Critical Thinking and Writing for Nursing Students (2nd Ed)
Evidence-based Practice in Nursing (2nd Ed)
Information Skills for Nursing Students
Reflective Practice in Nursing (2nd Ed)
Succeeding in Essays, Exams & OSCEs for Nursing Students
Succeeding in Literature Reviews and Research Project Plans for Nursing Students (2nd Ed)
Successful Professional Portfolios for Nursing Students (2nd Ed)
Understanding Research for Nursing Students (2nd Ed)

MENTAL HEALTH NURSING TITLES:

Assessment and Decision Making in Mental Health Nursing
Engagement and Therapeutic Communication in Mental Health Nursing
Medicines Management in Mental Health Nursing
Mental Health Law in Nursing
Physical Healthcare and Promotion in Mental Health Nursing
Psychosocial Interventions in Mental Health Nursing

ADULT NURSING TITLES:

Acute and Critical Care in Adult Nursing
Caring for Older People in Nursing
Medicines Management in Adult Nursing
Nursing Adults with Long Term Conditions
Safeguarding Adults in Nursing Practice
Dementia Care in Nursing

You can find more information on each of these titles and our other learning resources at **www.sagepub.co.uk**. Many of these titles are also available in various e-book formats, please visit our website for more information.

Foreword

The interplay between physical and mental health cannot be understated. This book provides us with a great opportunity to see both sides in action, to see how many physical ailments are influenced by, or even apparent symptoms of, mental health issues and vice versa. Traditionally, in healthcare, we have become blinkered in our thinking; body and mind somehow became separated and seen as disparate entities that had little influence over each other. This truly holistic book shows us ample examples of research and practice that prove this perspective to be flawed and helps the reader to consider aspects of both physical and mental health as one and same.

This book offers many practical suggestions as to how to ensure we successfully manage the physical healthcare needs of those in our care, underpinned by a broad base of theory and evidence. The principles of person centred recovery, validation, respect and dignity are themes that are interwoven throughout the chapters. The book provides practical exercises that will help the reader to develop a stronger understanding of the red flags we must notice in terms of physical health and helps us to think beyond the symptoms to the person experiencing them.

There is one outstanding theme, however, that bears further consideration as you embark on reading this text. The importance of a healthy lifestyle is a recurring theme throughout the chapters. It is essential that we are aware of our own lifestyle and remember that we are often seen as role models in caring for others, so caring for our own physical health is essential. The importance of good diet, exercise and sleep are repeatedly highlighted as essential for optimal health. There are some simple measures that a person can take to have substantial impact on their physical health that have been shown, in research, to have significant gains in terms of mental health too. The importance of this theme cannot be underestimated. The useful inclusion of models for change within the book helps to provide ideas about how we might go about educating and empowering others.

If you are a student nurse, a newly qualified nurse or even a nurse of some years' standing looking for tips to update your portfolio of skills, this book will stand you in good stead for practice. It can be read as a whole but can also be dipped into section by section as you come across situations in practice, perhaps, that warrant further exploration of that particular subject. Engaging with this book will help you to become a more effective practitioner of the art of mental health nursing, enhancing your ability to care for people of diverse backgrounds and needs.

Sandra Walker
Senior Teaching Fellow in Mental Health
University of Southampton

Acknowledgements

The author and publishers thank the following for permission to reproduce copyright material:

Häggström, M, Medical gallery of Mikael Häggström 2014. *Wikiversity Journal of Medicine*, for material reproduced as Figures 2.9, 7.3, 7.4 and 7.6.

Julius R, Novitsky M, Dubin W, Medication adherence: a review of the literature and implications for cllinical practice. *Journal of Psychiatric Practice*, 1 Jan 2009, Wolters Kluwer Health, for material reproduced as Table 3.1, Stages of change and associated patient characteristics and possible interventions.

Naranjo CA, Busto U, Sellers EM, Sandor P, Ruiz I *et al.* (1981) A method for estimating the probability of adverse drug reactions. *Clin. Pharmacol. Ther.*, 1 August, **30** (2), Nature Publishing Group, for material reproduced as Table 8.1, The adverse drug reaction scale.

Prochaska JO, DiClemente CC (1984) Self change processes, self efficacy and decisional balance across five stages of smoking cessation. *Prog. Clin. Biol. Res.* **156,** 131–140, for The process of change, reproduced as Figure 3.1.

The Rehabilitation for Addicted Prisoners Trust (RAPt) and Peter Gould ©, for material on disorders caused by alcohol, reproduced as Figure 7.2.

Smolensky M, Lamberg L (2000) *The Body Clock Guide to Better Health*, Henry Holt, for the human circadian (24-hour) biological clock, reproduced as Figure 2.4.

Finally, thank you to Simon Thistle for his artistic contribution.

About the author

Stan Mutsatsa PhD, RMN has extensive experience of working in both clinical and research settings in the nursing field of mental health. He has worked as a Research Associate at Imperial College for many years before taking up a post as Course Leader in Medication Management and later as a Physical Health Advisor on a large research project in physical health promotion, at Kings Institute of Psychiatry in London. Currently he is a Senior Lecturer in mental health nursing at City University London.

Introduction

Who is this book for?

This book aims to support pre-registration mental health nursing students to meet the Nursing and Midwifery Council (NMC) competencies in physical healthcare, including nursing practice and decision making, nutrition and fluid management, care, compassion and communication and medicines management from a recovery model perspective. It aims to prepare the student for a formative and summative assessment for entry into the register as a mental health nurse. Although the book is primarily aimed at nursing students at the pre-registration level of training, it is hoped that the book will serve as a useful reference guide for registered nurses. The link between theory and practice is explicit and the book is written in a style that is accessible and offers the correct academic challenge without diluting academic integrity.

Following the Chief Nursing Officer's report (Brimblecombe 2006) that called for mental health nurses to widen their skill base to include better skills to improve service users' physical well-being, the NMC published *Standards for Pre-registration Nursing* (2010) and Essential Skills Clusters (ESC) in line with the report's recommendations. This book fulfils some of the identified deficit in knowledge and skills at the point of registration.

This book is clearly linked to ESCs and will specifically cover the knowledge and skills required to be proficient in physical healthcare and promotion from a recovery approach perspective. It is a comprehensive textbook for student nurses undertaking the mental health nursing pathway, although it will also be useful for those undertaking other branches of nursing. It aims to prepare the student nurse for formative and summative assessments and also to meet the specific needs of this branch. It covers key topics such as the assessment of physical health; the therapeutic alliance and health beliefs; the effect of psychotropic medication on physical health; and the effects of substance misuse, metabolic syndrome, diabetes, exercise and diet. The book is practice-centred and encourages the student to be reflective through the use of case studies, scenarios and activities.

Why *Physical Healthcare and Promotion in Mental Health Nursing*?

There is suffcent evidence suggesting that people with mental health disorders suffer disproportionately from specific physical illnesses, including coronary heart disease, diabetes, infections, respiratory disease and also obesity. In many instances, the physical illness can be a direct result of the adverse effects of psychotropic medication. More importantly, available evidence shows that those with mental health problems are likely to have their physical health needs go unmet and are less likely to be offered checks on blood pressure, cholesterol, urine or weight, or to receive opportunistic advice on smoking cessation, alcohol, exercise or diet. In recognition of

1

these problems, the National Skills Framework (Department of Health 1999b) and the National Institute for Health and Care Excellence (NICE) emphasise the importance of good physical health in people with severe mental illness and encourage primary and secondary care services to collaborate to improve physical health outcomes in this population (NICE 2008).

Book structure

Chapter 1 looks at important factors known to influence physical health, such as lifestyle, treatment, illness-related and socio-cultural factors. Within the lifestyle concept, factors such as exercise, diet, smoking and the use of illicit drugs are discussed in more detail. With regard to treatment factors, the role of therapeutic drugs in worsening physical health, such as weight gain and adverse side effects, will be discussed.

Other issues covered are social class, poverty, unemployment and social inclusion.

Chapter 2 covers the assessment of physical health in people with mental health problems. The concept of wellness and homeostasis within the health context is discussed. General appearance, baseline vital signs, oxygen pulse, oxygen, respiration, blood pressure, peak flow and other physical health measures are discussed and the importance of each assessment and procedure is explained.

Chapter 3 covers the popular health theories that underpin health promotion. These include the Health Belief Model, the Self-Regulatory Model, Theory of Reasoned Action and the Five Stages of Change Model.

Chapter 4 initially gives an overview of the prevalence of cardiovascular illness in people with mental health problems. The chapter also covers the following subtopics: anatomy and physiology of the cardiovascular system, risk factors for cardiovascular health, disorders of the cardiovascular system, assessment of disorders, care and management of people with cardiovascular disorders, hypertension, hypotension, and preventive and health promotion.

Chapter 5 covers respiratory illness common in people with serious mental illness. The chapter includes prevalence of respiratory problems in mental illness, anatomy and physiology of the respiratory system, causes of respiratory illness, the effects of smoking, disorders of the respiratory system, assessment of respiratory disorders, care and management of people with respiratory disorders, preventive care and physical health promotion.

Chapter 6 covers diabetes and metabolic syndrome in mental health. Sections cover the prevalence of metabolic syndrome and diabetes in people with mental health disorders, anatomy and physiology of diabetes, causes of diabetes and metabolic syndrome, care and management of people with diabetes, preventive care and physical health promotion.

Chapter 7 covers misuse of substances in mental health and gives an overview of the prevalence of mental health problems in people who use psychoactive substances. The chapter covers the effects of alcohol and drugs such as cocaine, cannabis, heroin, amphetamines and tobacco on physical and mental health. Care management and health promotion are discussed.

Chapter 8 discusses the role of psychotropic medication in the physical health of those with mental health problems. The chapter focuses on key psychotropic side effects and their mechanism of action that are common to the treatment of mental health disorders. These side effects include extrapyramidal side effects, haematological and endocrinological side effects. Care and management of these side effects are discussed.

Chapter 9 discusses the role of nutrition and exercise in both physical and mental health. In particular, the role of exercise in alleviating conditions such as cardiovascular illness, cancer, depression, anxiety and schizophrenia is discussed. Further, the chapter discusses the role of nutrition and sleep hygiene in general health.

Requirements for the NMC Standards for Pre-registration Nursing Education and the Essential Skills Clusters

The NMC has established standards of competence to be met by applicants to different parts of the register, and these are the standards it considers necessary for safe and effective practice. In addition to the competencies, the NMC has set out specific skills that nursing students must be able to perform at various points of an education programme. These are known as ESCs. This book is structured so that it will help you to understand and meet the competencies and ESCs required for entry to the NMC register. The relevant competencies and ESCs are presented at the start of each chapter so that you can clearly see which ones the chapter addresses. This book includes the latest standards for 2010 onwards, taken from *Standards for Pre-registration Nursing* (NMC 2010).

Learning features

Activities

Throughout the book you will find activities in the text that will help you to make sense of, and learn about, the material being presented by the author.

Some activities ask you to reflect on aspects of practice, or your experience of it, or the people or situations you encounter. *Reflection* is an essential skill in nursing, and it helps you to understand the world around you and often to identify how things might be improved. Other activities will help you develop key skills such as your ability to *think critically* about a topic in order to challenge received wisdom, or your ability to *research a topic and find appropriate information and evidence*, and to be able to make decisions using that evidence in situations that are often difficult and time-pressured. Finally, communication and working as part of a team are core to all nursing practice, and some activities will ask you to carry out *group activities* or think about your *communication skills* to help develop these.

All the activities require you to take a break from reading the text, think through the issues presented and carry out some independent study, possibly using the internet. Where appropriate, sample answers are presented at the end of each chapter, and these will help you to understand more fully your own reflections and independent study. Remember, academic study will always require independent work; attending lectures will never be enough to be successful on your programme, and these activities will help to deepen your knowledge and understanding of the issues under scrutiny and give you practice at working on your own.

You might want to think about completing these activities as part of your personal development plan (PDP) or portfolio. After completing the activity write it up in your PDP or portfolio in a section devoted to that particular skill, then look back over time to see how far you have developed. You can also do more of the activities for a key skill that you have identified a weakness in, which will help build your skill and confidence in this area.

Chapter 1
The determinants of poor physical health in people with mental health problems

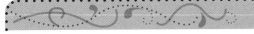
NMC Standards for Pre-registration Nursing Education

This chapter will address the following competencies:

Domain 3: Nursing practice and decision-making

Generic standard for competence
Nurses must practise autonomously, compassionately, skilfully and safely, and must maintain dignity and promote health and wellbeing. They must assess and meet the full range of essential physical and mental health needs of people of all ages who come into their care. Where necessary they must be able to provide safe and effective immediate care to all people prior to accessing or referring to specialist services irrespective of their field of practice. All nurses must also meet more complex and coexisting needs for people in their own nursing field of practice, in any setting including hospital, community and at home. All practice should be informed by the best available evidence and comply with local and national guidelines. Decision-making must be shared with service users, carers and families and informed by critical analysis of a full range of possible interventions, including the use of up-to-date technology. All nurses must also understand how behaviour, culture, socioeconomic and other factors, in the care environment and its location, can affect health, illness, health outcomes and public health priorities and take this into account in planning and delivering care.

NMC Essential Skills Clusters

This chapter will address the following ESCs:

Cluster: Care, compassion and communication
1. As partners in the care process, people can trust a newly registered graduate nurse to provide collaborative care based on the highest standards, knowledge and competence.
2. People can trust the newly registered graduate nurse to engage in person-centred care empowering people to make choices about how their needs are met when they are unable to meet them for themselves.

> ### Chapter aims
>
> By the end of the chapter, you should be able to:
>
> - understand the importance of physical health in people with mental health problems;
> - describe factors that influence poor physical health in people with mental health problems and how these factors interrelate.

Introduction

There is growing awareness through research that people with mental health disorders disproportionately suffer from specific physical health ailments. In particular those with severe mental illness (SMI), such as schizophrenia, depression or bipolar disorder, are at increased risk of suffering from cardiovascular disease (CVD), diabetes, infections, respiratory disease, cancer, infectious diseases and greater levels of obesity. In many others, weight gain is a clear side effect of psychotropic medication, particularly second-generation antipsychotics. People with SMI are almost twice as likely to die from coronary heart disease compared to the general population and four times more likely to die from respiratory disease (Brown *et al.* 1999; Nocon *et al.* 2004). In their analysis of records of 1.7 million primary care patients, the Disability Commission (2005) estimate that people with schizophrenia or bipolar disorder are more than twice as likely to have diabetes as other patients. In addition, they are more likely to experience **ischaemic** heart disease, stroke, hypertension and epilepsy compared to to the general population. Despite evidence of high prevalence of cardiovascular risk factors in this population, there is evidence of undertreatment of these modifiable risk factors. In an influential study, Clinical Antipsychotic Trials of Intervention Effectiveness (CATIE), 88% of patients with **dyslipidaemia**, 62% of those with **hypertension** and 38% of those with diabetes did not receive treatment for these ailments (Nasrallah *et al.* 2006a). This finding is in line with a large prospective study that has confirmed that many of these physical health problems are already present at the time of illness presentation (de Hert *et al.* 2006). A higher percentage of people with mental health problems use cannabis and other drugs than the general population (Boydell *et al.* 2006).

> ### Case study
>
> *Manesh is a 26-year-old man who suffers from bipolar disorder. He has had many previous admissions to hospital due to relapses in his condition. Periods of relapse coincide with heavy periods of cannabis use. During the winter months, he tends to suffer from a more severe and protracted form of chest infection. Coincidentally, he smokes more cannabis during the winter months.*

Regular cannabis use in people with SMI leads to increased relapse and hospitalisation. Moreover, cannabis use is associated with poor adherence to treatment and longer duration of illness (Grech *et al.* 2005; Kirsch *et al.* 2008). Patients who take cannabis are at increased risk of deterioration in physical health that includes bronchitis and lung cancer. Its use is highly prevalent in the UK and results in a vulnerability to SMI. A review of cannabis use in people with psychosis noted a misuse of 22.5% (Green *et al.* 2005).

There is evidence that people with mental health problems are disadvantaged by health inequalities and factors pertaining to these are complex and likely to include poverty, lifestyle, access to health assessments and treatments, and side effects of antipsychotic and mood-stabilising medication (Phelan *et al.* 2001).

A number of studies comparing people with mental health problems to the general population found that the former are less likely to be offered a number of interventions that include blood pressure, cholesterol, and urine or weight checks. In addition, they are less likely to receive opportunistic advice on smoking cessation, alcohol, exercise or diet (Phelan *et al.* 2001). As a nurse, you need to address this deficit actively to improve patient care.

Available evidence also shows that those with mental health problems are likely to have their physical health needs unattended to, unnoticed, poorly managed or simply dismissed as a reflection of their mental state. This underestimation of the significance of physical health problems because of significant psychiatric symptoms is called **diagnostic overshadowing**.

We see diagnostic overshadowing when we observe the high proportion of people with SMI not receiving tests assessing metabolic risk factors even for simple issues like obesity and blood pressure (Buckley *et al.* 2005). At present, neither mental health professionals nor primary healthcare professionals carefully screen or monitor patients receiving antipsychotic medication for metabolic risk factors (Hasnain *et al.* 2010). As an example of this problem, the CATIE schizophrenia study found non-treatment rates for diabetes in this population to be as high as 45.3%, in spite of clear National Institute for Health and Care Excellence guidelines (Nasrallah *et al.* 2006a). Undiagnosed diabetes and screening rates for metabolic abnormalities in people with SMI remain low, and may lead to prolonged periods of poor glycaemic control. As a nurse, you should pay greater attention at individual and system level to these physical disorders as they have the potential to reduce life expectancy and worsen psychiatric stability and treatment adherence, as well as quality of life.

Activity 1.1   *Critical thinking*

Melissa is a 46-year-old woman whose cancer was being treated with the medication interferon-alpha. After a few weeks of treatment, Melissa started to experience depressive symptoms and became suicidal. Her mood became so severe that one day she doused herself in oil and set herself alight. Fortunately, she survived.

continued . . .

What factors may have contributed to her low mood and how may these factors have been overlooked?

There are outline answers to all the activities at the end of the chapter.

Melissa's case is an example of how a patient's mental state can be overshadowed by the need to treat the underlying physical illness. In the next case study we see the effect of not paying enough attention to the physical health needs of people with SMI.

Case study

Jake is a 23-year-old man who has been suffering from schizophrenia since he was 18 years old. He is currently in hospital but generally keeps to himself and spends a lot of his time listening to music. He is prescribed olanzapine, which he takes regularly. One morning, he approached his primary nurse complaining of abdominal pain and increased urinary output. The primary nurse thought Jake was suffering from indigestion and gave him a dose of antacid. At lunchtime, Jake refused to eat his food, stating that he was not hungry, and continued to refuse food for the rest of that day, stating a lack of appetite. This was unusual for Jake.

The following day, Jake woke up much earlier than usual and had to be reminded to wash. He was irritable, raising his voice whilst talking to another patient, which was unusual for him. The nurse who attended to him was concerned about his behaviour and therefore offered Jake an extra dose of medication to help him to calm down, which he agreed to. An hour later Jake's physical condition deteriorated so dramatically that he was urgently transferred to a general hospital where he was diagnosed with a burst appendix.

As the case study demonstrates, the quality of physical healthcare provided to people with SMI is usually suboptimal. In Jake's case, if the nurse had asked further questions regarding his pain, it is likely that the nurse would have established that the pain was radiating around the umbilical region, that Jake had been vomiting and that his temperature was elevated. This extra information (symptoms of appendicitis) would have been very useful and provided sufficient reason for the healthcare team to take prompt action.

The nurse was quick to offer Jake PRN medication without further investigation; this is diagnostic overshadowing, which is a huge problem with negative health consequences for the patient. Jake was providing clear clues to the nurses that should have prompted further investigation: his irritability, late waking and refusal of food.

Attending to the physical health needs of people with SMI has been associated with multiple improvements in both mental and physical health, including improvement in self-esteem and well-being. Such multiple outcomes provide strong reasons for targeting support and treatment for people with SMI. In order to give this support, you need to understand the determinants of poor physical health in this client group.

This chapter starts by discussing the prevalence of long-term physical health problems in people with mental health problems in general and those with serious mental health problems in particular. It will then discuss specific factors that affect physical health problems in this population. Such factors can broadly be divided into lifestyle, treatment, biological, socio-economic and environmental factors. We will discuss lifestyle-related factors first.

Lifestyle-related factors

Case study

Owen is a 49-year-old man who has suffered from depression since he was 24. He has been a smoker since the age of 22. He smokes about 30 cigarettes a day. Recently, during an X-ray, the doctor noticed the presence of solitary small masses on his lungs, sometimes called **coin lesions**. *These lesions are consistent with the presence of lung cancer.*

We generally accept the view that lifestyle factors interact with biological factors to produce susceptibility to an illness. A lifestyle is a way of living that reflects the attitudes and values of a person or constellation of habitual activities unique to a person. Connolly and Kelly (2005) have asserted that a variety of factors, such as genes, environment and socio-demographic status, influence lifestyle. They further assert that, in schizophrenia, the illness itself contributes to shaping lifestyle. For example, people with schizophrenia tend to be unemployed and therefore drift down the social scale. This downward drift is usually associated with poorer financial standing and poor health. This view is supported by early studies that examined the effects of lifestyle factors on the physical health of people with schizophrenia living in the community (Brown *et al.* 1999; McCreadie 2003). These two studies compared the lifestyle factors of people with schizophrenia with that of low-social-class cohorts from the general population. In both studies, people with schizophrenia made significantly poorer dietary choices, took less exercise and smoked more than the general population. Before you read further, please take part in the activity below.

Activity 1.2   *Reflection*

The physical well-being of people with mental health problems is very important, but maintaining good physical health in this client group is generally poor. What is the best approach to care that has the potential to maximise physical well-being?

Smoking has emerged as one of the most potent factors of poor health in people with mental health problems. In comparison to the general population, people suffering from mental illness are at least twice as likely to smoke cigarettes. Approximately 80% of those with schizophrenia smoke cigarettes (McNeil 2001). The case study of Owen shows the problem of smoking and its complications. Higher rates of smoking have been observed in people suffering from other mental health problems, such as post-traumatic stress disorder (PTSD), according to an early systematic review (Fu *et al.* 2007). The review concluded that those exposed to traumatic events have higher smoking rates than those without such exposure. This systematic review of 45 studies found the prevalence of smoking to be as high as 80% in people suffering from PTSD (Fu *et al.* 2007). Moreover, observational studies indicate that smokers with PTSD have lower quit rates than those without PTSD.

Other studies have found that those with PTSD are particularly susceptible to the use of alcohol (Reynolds *et al.* 2005). PTSD provides a clear example of the interaction between illness type and lifestyle factors that have negative impacts on a person's physical health. In relation to other illnesses, nicotine dependence has a link with an increase in rates of depression before and after taking up smoking. It is also related to increased rates of suicidal ideation (Hughes 2008). In the case study, it is possible that Owen's depression may worsen because of his prolonged smoking and smoking may also have played a major role in the development of cancer.

A major factor that has an association with poor physical health is sedentary lifestyle. It has been reported that people with SMI are more likely to lead an inactive life than the general population (Brown *et al.* 1999). This sedentary lifestyle may be due to the sedating effect of most psychotropic medications or because of the negative symptoms that some people with SMI tend to suffer from. Evidently, this poses important problems as these people are likely to be at high risk of chronic medical conditions associated with inactivity. In particular, inactivity tends to put people at risk from obesity, which may lead to disorders like type 2 diabetes, hypertension, stroke and heart problems. Obesity due to inactivity is also linked to various cancers, including colon, breast, prostate and lung cancers (Pearce and Cheetham 2010).

Other lifestyle factors that may compromise physical health in people with mental health disorders is the use of alcohol and drugs. Before you read further, try the activity below.

Activity 1.3   *Critical thinking*

Ted, a 33-year-old male who suffers from schizophrenia and has a history of injecting heroin, is admitted to your ward. A few hours after admission, you notice that Ted is restless and the next day he complains of hearing derogatory voices. He also complains of muscle and bone pain, insomnia, diarrhoea, vomiting, cold flashes with goosebumps and leg movements. Can you identify factors that may have led to Ted's deteriorating physical and mental health?

The abuse of alcohol has a relationship with multiple physical problems, including cancer, digestive system problems, liver disease, cardiovascular problems, and both central and peripheral nervous system problems. In addition to alcohol usage, people with mental health problems and SMI in particular use cannabis more than the general population. This disproportionate use of cannabis leads to physical ailments affecting cardiac, vascular and respiratory function. Further, the use of psychoactive substances in people with SMI worsens their psychiatric symptoms, as in the case of Ted above. This view is supported by an early longitudinal study that followed up 152 people with first-episode schizophrenia. At follow-up, persistent substance users had significantly more severe positive symptoms and depressive symptoms and greater overall severity of illness (Harrison *et al.* 2008). In a recent study of people with no previous history of depression, the investigators found depressive symptoms were associated with an increase in rates of self-reported opioid misuse (Grattan *et al.* 2012). As part of effective nursing care, it is important that you assess your patients for the use of psychoactive substances.

Another important aspect of lifestyle that impacts on poor physical health in people with mental health problems is dietary intake. In general, the western lifestyle is characterised by the consumption of high-energy foods rich in fat, refined carbohydrates and animal protein. This, in combination with the tendency for low physical activity that is common in many western societies, leads to an overall energy imbalance. This imbalance has a strong association with a multitude of health disorders that include obesity, diabetes, CVD, arterial hypertension and cancer. People with mental health problems are at an elevated risk of developing these metabolic-related disorders partly due to poor dietary choices.

It has been previously reported that people who suffer from SMI tend to have poor dietary habits, and one of the early studies to examine this relationship was carried out by McCreadie (2003). In a cross-sectional study, the investigator examined the dietary habits of 104 community-dwelling people with schizophrenia. The author found that, compared to the general population, males with SMI consumed significantly less fruit, vegetables, milk, potatoes and pulses. Significantly fewer females consumed milk and potatoes compared with the general population. This early important finding is supported by another early study by Peet (2004), among others. A higher dietary intake of refined sugar and dairy products was predictive of a worse 2-year outcome of schizophrenia. A low dietary intake of fish and seafood was predictive of a high prevalence of depression.

These earlier findings have subsequently been replicated in more recent studies (Casagrande *et al.* 2011). A meta-analytic study of 31 studies concluded that people with schizophrenia tend to have a poor dietary pattern that partly accounts for their higher incidence of metabolic abnormalities (Dipasquale *et al.* 2013). Therefore, the poor dietary intake of people with mental health problems has important negative consequences on the physical health and recovery in this population. One important dietary factor that has a link to poor physical health in people with mental health problems is vitamin D deficiency, linked to a host of disorders, including diabetes, CVD, cancer and bone and muscle disorders. In addition, vitamin D deficiency is associated with psychiatric illness such as depression, anxiety and schizophrenia (see Chapter 9). Treatment factors contribute to poor physical health in people with mental health problems and we will turn our attention to these next.

Treatment-related factors

Case study

*Rajiv is a 45-year-old man of Caribbean origin. He suffers from bipolar disorder but his symptoms are well controlled by clozapine and lithium carbonate. He has been taking this medication regularly for 2 years but has gained weight. At 1.75 m (5 foot 9 inches), he now weighs 99 kg (220 lb) and smokes 20 cigarettes a day. Recently, he went to see his GP for a check-up. Though he considers himself to be in good physical health, the examination revealed the following. Blood pressure was 160/95 mmHg. His fasting blood sugar level was 8.9 mmol/L, haemoglobin A_{1C} 8.1%, cholesterol 6.85 mmol/L, high-density lipoprotein 0.91 mmol/L, low-density lipoprotein 4.78 mol/L, triglycerides 2.82 mmol/L and very-low-density lipoprotein 1.34 mmol/L. Results of liver and renal function tests were within the normal range. The urine was positive for albumin. The GP diagnosed Rajiv with **metabolic syndrome**. A low-calorie, low-sodium, cholesterol and carbohydrate diet was recommended by his GP, in addition to an exercise regimen.*

In addition to other factors, Rajiv's weight gain can be attributed to the use of psychotropic medication like clozapine and lithium. The use of psychotropic medication is among the most obvious and potent factors of poor physical health in people with mental health problems. These medications cause side effects and one notable side effect is weight gain. Weight can progress to obesity and this is usually accompanied by increase in body fat. Specifically, central or upper-body obesity has an association with dyslipidaemia, impaired glucose tolerance, insulin resistance, hypertension, heart problems, low blood pressure, osteoporosis and seizures.

Daumit and colleagues (2003) conducted a study that examined the level of obesity in people with SMI in the community and found that 29% of men and 60% of women were obese. In many cases, the contributory factor for this obesity is antipsychotic medication, as with Rajiv. For his condition, Rajiv takes clozapine and lithium carbonate: both medications have a propensity for causing weight gain. We see that, although Rajiv has not complained of any specific physical ailments, the results of his routine physical examination are worrying. From an economic perspective, Chwastiak *et al.* (2009) found that the healthcare costs for more than 1,400 individuals with schizophrenia who participated in an 18-month trial in the USA (Nasrallah *et al.* 2006b) were 25% higher for those who were obese. The investigators suggest that this figure is probably an underestimate of the true costs of treating obesity given the short timeframe of study. Clearly, there are many personal, social and economic consequences of obesity. Before you read further, please take part in the activity below.

Activity 1.4   *Evidence-based practice and research*

Make a note of Rajiv's blood test results and compare them with the normal ranges of blood pressure, fasting blood sugar, haemoglobin A_{1C} and cholesterol.

In addition to weight gain, antipsychotic medication can induce a variety of physical ill effects, including constipation, blurred vision, drowsiness, blood disorders and movement disorders (see Chapter 8). These movement disorders include parkinsonism, dystonia and akathisia. Hormonal side effects are equally common with the use of psychotropics. A key physical health risk factor in the use of antipsychotic medication is the development of insulin resistance via dyslipidaemia. **Hyperlipidaemia** may develop and this may be independent of weight increase in a patient. A recent systematic review compared risperidone and other antipsychotics on a range of outcomes and concluded that risperidone seems to produce more hormonal and extrapyramidal side effects than most second-generation antipsychotics or atypicals. The authors also reported that adverse effects have an impact on a patient's physical health, such as cardiometabolic problems, sedation and seizures (Komossa *et al.* 2011). In practice, both lifestyle and treatment factors interact with intrinsic biological factors to induce physical health problems and we will turn to these next.

Biological factors

Case study

Peter, a 48-year-old male of African-Caribbean origin, visited his GP with a 5-day history of nausea and vomiting. He also reported a 2-week history of excessive passing of urine (polyuria) and excessive thirst (polydipsia) and a 5-kg weight loss. His GP conducted a physical examination which showed an **afebrile**, *obese man (body mass index 40 kg/m²) with prominent hyperpigmentation of the skin (acanthosis nigricans). Laboratory blood tests showed Peter had* **metabolic acidosis**, *and* **hyperglycaemia** *(pH 7.14, bicarbonate 6 mmol/L, urinary ketones 8.3 mmol/L and glucose 11 mmol/L). He also informed his GP that his older sister suffers from diabetes and believed that his maternal grandmother had a similar condition. He was diagnosed with type 2 diabetes.*

Metabolic syndrome and diabetes

It is well known that conditions such as cardiovascular illness, diabetes, obesity and hypetension have a genetic basis and therefore are inheritable. With regard to type 2 diabetes, available evidence suggests that this condition clusters in specific ethnic minority groups such as those from the Indian subcontinent, parts of Latin America, and in people of African and Caribbean origin. The case study of Peter above is a case in point. It is also known that type 2 diabetes has many causes, with subtypes that have a strong association with environmental factors at one end of the spectrum and highly genetic forms at the other end (Froguel *et al.* 2000). Genes responsible for type 2 diabetes have largely been isolated and include those responsible for **glucokinase**, and four transcription factors (proteins that bind to specific DNA sequences, thereby controlling the flow of genetic information from DNA), which play a key role in the development of the endocrine pancreas or in the expression of glucose metabolism genes. A recent systematic review of literature that examined the early onset of type 2 diabetes across ethnicities found populations with Amerindian or African heritages to have the highest prevalence of diabetes worldwide (Irving *et al.* 2011). In countries such as Mexico and Jamaica (Peter's origin), where diabetes is highly prevalent, the onset of the disease is earlier, usually before the age of 40. The review also found that two-thirds of the early-onset diabetes cases studied have a body mass index over 25 kg/m^2 and that the clinical characteristics of metabolic syndrome were present. Furthermore, they found that a minority of these patients had mutations in the **maturity-onset diabetes of the young** (MODY) genes. People from these ethnic backgrounds are overrepresented within the mental health system. In reality, these patients are likely to be prescribed psychotropic medication, therefore compounding the risk of developing not only diabetes but also cardiovascular disorders.

Heart disease

Cardiovascular conditions that are common in people with SMI are not only genetically influenced but are also gender-specific. In the general population, CVD is the leading cause of mortality in women. In fact, CVD accounts for a third of all deaths of women worldwide and 50% of all female mortality over 50 years of age in developing countries (Pilote *et al.* 2007). Retrospective studies suggest there is a clear difference between men and women in terms of prevalence, presentation, management and outcomes of the disease. For instance, women who suffer from diabetes have a significantly higher CVD mortality rate than men with diabetes. Similarly, women with **atrial fibrillation** are at greater risk of stroke than men with this condition. Over the last decades, mortality rates in men with CVD have steadily declined, while those in women have remained stable.

The mechanism underlying these gender-specific differences is subject to investigation, but we believe that genetic factors play an important part. The advent of **genome-wide association studies** has created significant advances in our knowledge of the link between CVD and genetics. Currently, at least gene positions on a chromosome map associated with CVD and its risk factors have been identified (Arking and Chakravarti 2009). In people with SMI, genetic factors are likely to interact with lifestyle and treatment factors, therefore significantly compounding the risk of CVD. For example, cardiac arrhythmias have a genetic base and many psychotropic medications like olanzapine are known to cause cardiac arrhythmias. Together, these two factors synergistically increase the risk of developing cardiac problems in people with SMI. As with CVD, cancers are very common in people with SMI.

Cancers

In general, cancer rates are set to increase at an alarming rate globally, emerging as a major public health problem in developing countries similar to its impact in industrialized nations. In 2003, the World Health Organization (WHO) estimated that different types of cancer account for 12.6% of global deaths yearly. The report also predicts that cancers will increase by 50% to 15 million new cases a year by 2020. This predicted sharp increase in new cases will mainly be due to a steady increase in ageing populations worldwide, current trends in smoking prevalence and the growing adoption of unhealthy lifestyles.

In people with mental health problems and those with SMI in particular, the environmental and lifestyle factors (smoking, unhealthy diet, drinking alcohol) contribute significantly to the prevalence of cancer, but, as in the general population, genetic factors play an important part. For example, prostate and breast cancers are known to be familial (Shen and Abate-Shen 2010), while lifestyle factors like alcohol consumption and sedentary lifestyle significantly increase the risk for breast and prostate cancer (Laamiri *et al.* 2014). In this respect, it is important for you as a nurse to enquire from the patient about a family history and lifestyle during assessment.

In addition to the factors so far described, socio-economic factors can significantly influence poor physical health in people with mental health problems.

Socio-economic factors

In many societies most diseases are more common further down the social ladder (Wilkinson and Marmot 2003). Poorer people usually have twice the risk of serious illness and premature death compared to those near the top of the social scale. Stressful life circumstances that make people worried, anxious or unable to cope are damaging and can lead to premature death; these are more common in poorer people. These psychosocial risks accumulate during the course of a person's life and they exert a powerful effect on both the physical and mental health of an individual. Long periods of anxiety and insecurity or a lack of supportive friendship is detrimental. The further down on the social ladder people are, the more prevalent these problems (Wilkinson and Marmot 2003). Poorer people tend to receive healthcare that is generally poorer in quality than those who are wealthy. According to the WHO report (2008a), this maldistribution of healthcare is responsible for appalling premature loss of life which arises principally because of the conditions in which people are born, grow, live, work and age. According to Marmot (2004), poor and unequal living conditions are, in their turn, a result of deeper structural conditions that together shape the way societies are organised (e.g. poor social policies and programmes, unfair economic arrangements and bad politics). In this regard you need to develop an awareness of people's social and economic conditions and how these affect their health. You will notice that most people with mental health problems and SMI in particular are likely to be unemployed and this pushes them further down the social hierarchy. Not surprisingly, they are likely to suffer financial contraints that will impact on their ability to sustain themselves adequately in terms of affording the right types of food or housing and this will ultimately have a bearing on their physical and mental health.

Research into the effects of unemployment on physical and mental health has been consistent (Linn *et al.* 1985; Turner 1995). Linn *et al.* (1985) compared data of two groups of men who were unemployed with those who were employed. They found that those who were unemployed complained of somatic symptoms, including depression and anxiety, more than in the employed group. More importantly, they found that those who were unemployed made significantly more visits to their doctor, took more medications and spent more days in bed sick than did employed individuals. Since many people suffering from mental health problems tend to be unemployed, findings from this study can be extrapolated in this population.

Further, this is in keeping with Wilkinson and Marmot's (2003) finding that it is in fact the social and economic conditions that trigger and foster ill health. They have also asserted that, as social beings, we need not only good material conditions, but from childhood onwards, we also need to be valued and appreciated. We need to have friends, feel useful and exercise a certain degree of control over our work. Without these, we become more prone to depression, drug abuse, hostility and feelings of hopelessness, and these all rebound on physical health. Despite the obvious need for people with mental health problems to be valued and needed, these people are quite likely to go without employment, to be poor, socially excluded or suffer stigma, and this has a profound negative effect on their health.

Clearly the social determinants of physical health cannot be overstimated. In reality these factors have a close link to environmental factors.

Environmental factors

Exposure to ambient air pollution is a serious health concern, with an association with growing morbidity and mortality worldwide. In the last decades, research has established the adverse effects of air pollution on the pulmonary and cardiovascular systems. People who suffer from mental health problems tend to live in urban settings where pollution is prevalent and therefore are at risk of developing some of these physical illnesses. Furthermore, air pollution has also been associated with diseases of the central nervous system (CNS), including stroke, Alzheimer's disease, Parkinson's disease and neurodevelopmental disorders. It has been demonstrated that extremely small particles can easily translocate to the CNS, where they can activate innate immune responses. Systemic inflammation arising from the pulmonary or cardiovascular system can affect CNS health and emerging evidence suggests that air pollution induces neuroinflammation, **oxidative stress**, microglial activation, cerebrovascular dysfunction and alterations in the blood–brain barrier which will contribute to CNS disorders. This situation is likely to be reflected in people with mental health problems. Overall, socio-environmental factors play a significant role in the physical health of people with mental health problems.

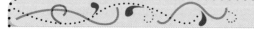

Chapter summary

Research evidence suggests that people with SMI have an excess mortality that is two or three times higher than in the general population. This mortality gap has widened in recent decades, even in countries where the quality of the healthcare system is good. About 60% of this excess mortality is due to physical illness. In particular, it is known that people with mental health problems experience physical health problems such as diabetes, CVD and many others. The possible reasons for this are that many people with mental health problems also suffer exposure to a variety of risk factors that can be can broadly categorised as lifestyle, treatment, biological and socio-economic. People with serious mental illness in particular are less likely to exercise and more likely to drink alcohol, smoke, take drugs and to have unhealthy eating habits. In addition, they are likely to be unemployed and there-fore are lower down on the social ladder. More importantly, these people are likely to suffer from a range of ailments as a result of treatment with psychotropic medi-cation. This renders them vulnerable to a range of physical and psychiatric illness. Like the general population, people with serious mental illness are also biologically vulnerable to certain physical illnesses such as cancer, diabetes and cardiovascular dieseases. Clearly, poor physical health in people with mental health problems is a serious public health challenge and one which also needs to be addressed in your own nursing care of your patients.

Activities: brief outline answers

Activity 1.1

There are two key factors in why Melissa was so depressed. The first is the nature of the illness she was suffering from. Even though the treatment and prognosis of cancer have improved over the years, in many instances cancer is still regarded as a terminal illness and this imposes a huge psychological burden on the sufferer. Second, the drug interferon-alpha is known to induce depression and this could most likely have added to the psychological burden imposed by the illness.

Activity 1.2

One proposed appraoch is to use a life-course approach that promotes a positive start in life and healthy adult and older years. A life-course approach typically starts from the perinatal stage of development until old age. Integrating physical and mental health is important in promoting a whole-person approach that reduces the health-risk behaviour and enhances physical activity.

Activity 1.3

Ted's symptoms are consistent with withdrawal symptoms of heroin. Apart from the agreed care, you should consider assessing Ted with a view to implementing a drug withdrawal programme based on recovery principles, including empowering the individual and respect. Before you do this, you need to confirm Ted is suffering from drug withdrawal symptoms and the best way to do this is to test for the presence of drugs in his urine.

Activity 1.4

Fasting blood sugar: 4.4–6.1 mmol/L

Haemoglobin A_{1C}: 4–6%

Cholesterol: 3.5–6.5 mmol/L (ideally, levels should be below 5 mmol/L)

Further reading

Department of Health (2011) *Healthy Lives, Healthy People: A call to action on obesity in England.* London: DoH.

This document sets out how the new approach to public health will enable effective action on obesity and encourages a wide range of partners to play their part.

Useful websites

http://www.who.int/social_determinants/en

This is a very useful WHO website with information on determinants of health.

http://www.who.int/hia/evidence/doh/en/index3.html

Another WHO website that has information on different determinants of health.

http://www.dh.gov.uk/prod_consum_dh/groups/dh_digitalassets/documents/digitalasset/dh_126449.pdf

This document sets out the Department of Health's 3-year social marketing strategy for changing health-related lifestyle behaviours and improving health outcomes.

Chapter 2
The physical health assessment in mental health nursing

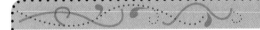

Chapter aims

By the end of the chapter, you should be able to:

- understand the principle of homeostasis and how it relates to the physical health–mental health balance;
- understand the theoretical concepts underpinning common physical health assessments;
- undertake common physical health assessments.

Introduction

Case study

Stuart is a 51-year-old unemployed man who has used mental health services for 25 years. He was diagnosed with schizophrenia but he lives independently with the support of his family and a care coordinator. His physical health is generally good but he was seen recently by his GP, who recorded Stuart's weight as 85 kg (body mass index (BMI) 32 kg/m²), blood pressure (BP) 150/95 mmHg and total cholesterol 7.5 mmol/L. Stuart smokes 15–20 cigarettes daily, drinks around 25 units of alcohol per week and does not exercise. Stuart's diet consists largely of ready-made meals and he eats relatively little freshly prepared food.

In 1857, Claude Bernard suggested that the internal environment is the condition for life. We call this internal condition homeostasis, and its definition is *the ability or tendency of an organism to maintain internal equilibrium by adjusting its physiological processes.* If we consider the case of Stuart above, we can note that Stuart's BP is 150/95 mmHg, which is above normal (120/80 mmHg). From a homeostatic point of view, Stuart's high BP reflects a lack of balance in his body's internal environment (we will discuss this in more detail later) and treatment is therefore necessary to restore internal equilibrium.

As we discussed in Chapter 1, people with mental health problems concurrently suffer from physical health disorders brought about by a disturbance of their internal environment (homeostasis). We can easily argue that Stuart's homeostasis is disturbed and therefore in need of correction. Before we can correct the internal environment (homeostasis), we need to assess the level of disturbance of the internal environment. The most common way of doing this is to carry out a physical health assessment, as Stuart's doctor did. This chapter will start by discussing the concept of homeostasis as a basis for understanding physical health assessment. The chapter then discusses the biological aspects underlying each particular assessment before outlining practical procedures for each physical health assessment. In particular, the chapter covers the assessment of baseline vital signs, oxygen, pulse, respiration, BP, peak flow, electrocardiogram (ECG), BMI and weight circumference ratio. We now turn our attention to homeostasis.

The concept of homeostasis

As previously mentioned, many diseases and disorders result from a disturbance of the internal environment, known as homeostatic imbalance. Rinomhota and Cooper (1996) suggest that, for life to continue, successful regulation of homeostasis in necessary. In other words, our body has to reach a 'steady state' that resists change from outside forces to function optimally. We commonly refer to this steady state as **dynamic equilibrium**. Thus, homeostasis is not static but dynamic, in continuous change, yet where relatively uniform conditions prevail. For example, if Stuart's BP is measured three times at different times and after performing exercises and the reading remains close to 150/95 mmHg, we can say his BP is in a steady state or dynamic equilibrium.

Disruption of the steady-state condition can result in discomfort, illness, disease or death. This is because, when the body fails to regulate or maintain a steady-state internal environment, toxins accumulate in the body, and this leads to the destruction of cells and tissues (Rinomhota and Cooper 1996). More importantly, as our body ages, it loses efficiency in its regulatory system and this will ultimately result in an unstable internal environment which in turn increases the risk for illness.

So what causes homeostasis? The nervous system regulates homeostasis in the short term and the endocrine system in the long term. We feel the effects of the nervous system, such as the control of body temperature, within minutes. If you enter a hot place, your body will start producing sweat as a way of regulating your body temperature and this may happen within minutes of entering. By contrast, homeostatic regulation by the endocrine system may take hours, days or weeks to take effect. This is because the endocrine system exerts its effect through the production of hormones which travel to their target organ or place of action via the blood. As a result, the endocrine system is often slow in producing its effects. A typical example is the production of insulin after eating a meal rich in carbohydrates to assist in regulating blood sugar levels in the body. To take effect, this process can take hours. Overall, homeostasis is an integrated enterprise that involves both the endocrine and the nervous systems. It is essential for the survival of cells and, therefore, our body. Before you read further, please take part in the activity below.

Activity 2.1	Critical thinking

In a group or on your own, make a list of conditions or physical illness common in people with mental health problems that could be a result of poor regulation of the internal environment.

There are outline answers to all the activities at the end of the chapter.

Swanson (1991) suggests that you should not regard the concept of homeostasis as purely biological and something to learn within a classroom. Instead, you should link these concepts with your daily nursing activities. For this reason, we will discuss the role of temperature regulation from a homeostatic perspective before we discuss the practical aspects of temperature measurement.

Temperature and its measurement

Case study

It was mid-August and Jenny was on holiday in Spain with her 84-year-old mother Margaret, who had just recovered from a bout of depression. For the first week of their holiday, the temperature was above 42°C. One particularly hot sunny day, Jenny left her mother in the holiday apartment to attend to some errands. When she returned at midday, she found her mother unconscious on the sofa in the living room. All the windows were closed. Jenny tried to rouse her mother but Margaret could say only a few words and she seemed delirious. Jenny called for help and the emergency services operator instructed her to apply cold flannels to her mother's forehead and face and to position her mother in front of a fan while using a spray bottle to spray lukewarm water on her skin.

When the paramedics arrived Margaret was conscious but confused and feeling nauseous. At the hospital, the doctor told Jenny that her mother had suffered heat stroke, a form of hyperthermia, and that it was Jenny's quick action at the house that had saved her mother's life.

The regulation of body temperature and measurement

The regulation of body temperature, thermoregulation, is the ability of the body to keep its body temperature within certain limits irrespective of the environmental temperature. The part of the brain which regulates the body's ability to maintain a constant body temperature is the hypothalamus (Mutsatsa 2011), which is rich in neurons sensitive to cold and heat that monitor blood temperature as the blood passes through. The impulse firing rate of the heat-sensitive neurons increases as the temperature of the body increases. Margaret's heat-sensitive neurons in the hypothalamus were firing rapidly because of heat stroke.

The body metabolism maintains a core or deep body temperature of 37.1°C, which varies slightly from person to person and time of day. There are many sites where you can measure core temperature and each site has a range of normal temperatures. For example, the oral-site temperature tends to vary between 36.5 and 37.5°C. Furthermore, all types of temperature measurement have advantages and limitations that relate to accuracy, precision, practicality and feasibility in a clinical setting.

You should avoid taking temperature at the peripherals such as arms and legs, as it is unstable, and fluctuates rapidly. This is because environmental temperatures easily influence peripheral temperature. With respect to core temperature, there are several factors which influence its reading:

- Age: there is wide normal variation of temperatures in young children due to a less effective temperature-regulatory mechanism. In older adults, normal temperatures are usually lower than in other age groups and this is because the efficiency of homeostatic mechanism decreases with age, as was the case with Margaret. In the elderly, normal core temperatures tend to average around 36.2°C.

- Women of childbearing age: the secretion of the hormone progesterone at mid-cycle results in an increase in normal body temperature of 0.3–0.6°C.

- Exercise: in general, moderate to vigorous exercise increases normal body temperature.

- Diurnal cycle: during a 24-hour period, the normal body temperature fluctuates between 0.6°C and 0.9°C, with the highest body temperature occurring in the late afternoon and the lowest in the early-morning hours (see Figure 2.4, below).

Clearly, several factors influence body temperature and therefore it is important for you to integrate these important elements in core body temperature measurements. We can measure core body temperature using various routes, but the traditional route is the oral method. This is because it is accurate and convenient in spite of technological advances. Oral temperature closely approximates that of the carotid artery, which links intimately the temperature-regulatory centres of the hypothalamus. Therefore, measurement of oral temperature is more likely to reflect core temperature. The core body temperature is usually constant and is the only temperature at which vital organs such as the brain, heart and liver function optimally. Oral temperatures are generally about 0.4°C (0.9°F) lower than rectal temperatures. Drinking, chewing, smoking and breathing with the mouth open all influence oral temperature. For example, cold drinks or food reduce oral temperatures; hot drinks, hot food, chewing and smoking raise oral temperature (Kelly 2007).

Oral route

In taking oral temperature, you should place the thermometer under the tongue, at the base in either of the posterior sublingual pockets, and then instruct the person to keep the lips closed but not clamp the teeth.

Leave the thermometer in situ for at least 3 minutes if the person has no fever (afebrile) and take up to 8 minutes if the temperature is febrile before taking a reading. You may take other vital signs during this time. If your patient has just smoked a cigarette, you need to wait at least 2 minutes before taking temperature and wait 15 minutes if the patient has just drunk hot or iced liquids. In addition to the oral route, we use the rectal route in measuring core temperature and particularly where the oral route is inappropriate.

Rectal route

This route is a better approximation of a person's body temperature than the oral and axillary routes. In addition, it is better to use this route in conditions that contraindicate the oral route. Before you read further, please take part in the activity below.

Activity 2.2	*Critical thinking*

Can you think of situations in clinical practice where the use of oral-route temperature measurement might present problems?

In measuring rectal temperature, you should wear gloves and insert a lubricated rectal probe on a thermometer that is no more than 3 cm long into the adult rectum, directed towards the umbilicus. If it is a glass thermometer, you should leave it in situ for approximately 3 minutes. In general, rectal temperature ranges from 36 to 38°C and is 0.4–0.5°C higher than core temperature. You will need to deduct about 0.5°C from the reading you obtain to get a true reading of the body temperature. A particular disadvantage of the rectal route is that it causes patient discomfort and it is invasive. We now turn our attention to the axillary method of temperature measurement.

Axillary and tympanic membrane route

This route is usually safe and accurate, particularly in infants and those who are confused. Another increasingly popular method for the measurement of core temperature is the use of the tympanic membrane thermometer, and it is growing in popularity.

The tympanic membrane thermometer senses infrared emission from the tympanic membrane (eardrum) in detecting core temperature. The eardrum shares the same blood supply (internal carotid artery) as the hypothalamus, thus making it a good approximate of core temperature, although its precision is not as good as the rectal route (Lawson *et al.* 2007). However, the advantages of the tympanic membrane thermometer are that it is non-invasive, non-traumatic, safe, there is a low cross-infection risk and it is very quick and efficient. It is very suitable for use in the mental health setting where most patients are likely to experience cognitive problems.

In measuring temperature using this procedure, gently place the covered probe tip in the person's ear canal and activate the device. You will be able to read the digital temperature in approximately 3 seconds. During this procedure, you should take care not to force the probe into the canal or shut it.

We now turn to another equally important clinical assessment, which is the measurement of pulse.

Pulse measurement

The blood is extremely important to our survival because it is the body's own transport system. It transports water, oxygen, nutrients, hormones, waste and many other substances. Because blood is a liquid, it needs a pump to move it around and the heart performs this task (we will discuss this in more detail in later sections). The pumping action of the heart due to contraction of the left-side ventricle exerts pressure on the arterial walls. Pumping blood causes a momentary expansion of the blood vessel (artery). We record this momentary expansion as a pulse. In a normal adult, the pulse rate is about 72 beats/min. All arteries in the body demonstrate pulse, but not all are accessible for examination by feeling and pressing with the palms of the hands (palpation). There are

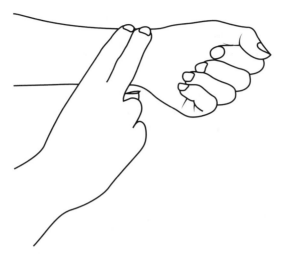

Figure 2.1: Taking your own pulse

many arterial pulse body sites and these include facial, temporal, brachial, carotid and radial. Traditionally, the radial pulse is mostly used and we find this on the inner aspect of the wrist (Blows 2012) (Figure 2.1). You should start the measurement of pulse by palpating, as Figure 2.1 shows.

Using the pad of your first two fingers, palpate the radial pulse at the flexor aspect of the wrist, laterally along the radius bone.

Push until you can feel the strongest pulsation and, if the rhythm is regular, count the number of beats for 30 seconds and then multiply by 2 to get the correct pulse rate per minute. In some instances, you could count the number of beats for 15 seconds and then multiply by 4, but this method is less accurate.

If the pulse rhythm is irregular, begin counting intervals with zero for the first pulse and one for the second pulse. You should continue counting for a full minute. In assessing the pulse, you should take account of the following: the rate, rhythm, strength and elasticity of the pulse.

The resting healthy adult has a pulse that ranges between 60 and 100 beats/min, depending on a number of factors that include age. Usually, the pulse is rapid during infancy, averaging 120 beats/min during the first year after birth, and is moderate in adults, averaging 75 beats/min for a healthy person. Males have slightly less rapid pulses than females after puberty. In normal well-trained athletes, the pulse is usually less than 60 beats/min. This is because their heart muscles are strong and well developed, able to push out a larger volume of blood at each beat, thus requiring fewer beats per minute to maintain a stable heart output. As a good example of an athlete with a low pulse rate, the French newspaper *L'Équipe* reported in 2004 that the professional cyclist Miguel Indurain had a resting pulse of 28 beats/min!

A pulse normally has an even pace, but from time to time irregularity occurs and we commonly find this in children and young adults. One such condition that shows irregularity is sinus arrhythmia. This is a condition where the pulse rate increases at the peak of inspiration and goes back to normal during expiration.

The force of a pulse normally indicates the strength of the heart stroke volume. If the pulse is weak and feels like a small cord or thread under the finger ('thready'), this is an indication of decreased stroke volume, which we normally associate with haemorrhage shock. A full bounding pulse may be an indication of increased stroke volume, as in the case of anxiety, exercise and some medical conditions. Additionally, there are abnormal pulse conditions that you may come across and the most common are bradycardia and tachycardia. Bradycardia is when the pulse rate falls below 60 beats/min. In this condition, the heart may not be pumping enough blood and this may result in fainting, shortness of breath, cardiac arrest or even death. We often consider resting bradycardia as normal if the individual has no accompanying symptoms such as fatigue, weakness, dizziness, light-headedness, fainting, chest discomfort, palpitations or shortness of breath.

When the pulse rate goes above 100 beats/min, we call this tachycardia. When the heart beats very fast, it pumps less efficiently and provides less blood to the rest of the body, including the heart itself. This increased work and limited oxygen supply can combine to form a heart ischaemia that is related to the pulse rate (Fauci *et al.* 2008). In some situations, the cause of tachycardia is high levels of anxiety and exercise.

In addition to pulse, respiration is another important physical health assessment and we will discuss this next.

Respiration

To gain an appreciation of a patient's oxygen delivery system, we need to understand how the respiratory system functions. This provides us with a wealth of information that relates to a patient's condition, be it respiratory, cardiovascular or neurological.

Respiration supplies the body's cells with oxygen and removes carbon dioxide, a byproduct of metabolism. The medulla, a part of the brain, acts as the respiratory centre that regulates breathing, an involuntary activity. We can divide the process of respiration into two phases: expiration and inspiration.

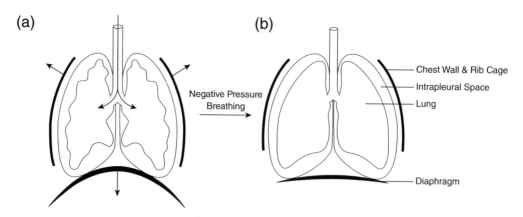

Figure 2.2: (a) The diaphragm elevated and the rib cage slightly contracting, causing positive pressure and resulting in air being expelled out of the lungs. (b) The diaphragm depressed and rib cage slightly expanded, causing negative pressure and resulting in airflow into the lungs

During expiration, as the lungs expel air that is replete with carbon dioxide and depleted in oxygen, the diaphragm moves upward and the rib cage contracts slightly, creating positive pressure in the rib cage, as Figure 2.2a shows. The creation of positive pressure forces air out of the lungs and this then leads to inspiration. During inspiration, the chest wall and rib cage expand and the diaphragm moves downward to a flat position (Figure 2.2b), creating a negative pressure inside the rib cage. This allows air replete in oxygen to flow inside the lungs. A series of diffusion mechanisms transports the oxygen to various parts of the body, where it takes part in biochemical processes.

In measuring respiration, you need to account for several factors that make up part of your respiration rate assessment. These factors are the rate, breath sounds, breathing effort, rhythm and depth of respiration.

In many cases, we can consider the respiration rate between 12 and 18 breaths/min as normal and we call this eupnoea. When the breathing rate exceeds 12 breaths/min, we call this tachypnoea. We call slow breathing that is less than 12 breaths/min bradypnoea. Breathing rate should normally have an even tempo but when there is an alteration to the rhythm and depth, it can be an indication of hyperventilation. Anxiety, fear, hepatic coma, neurological complications or alterations in the blood gas concentration can all be causes of hyperventilation. In some cases, we can observe Cheyne–Stokes respiration, characterised by progressively deeper and sometimes faster breathing. A gradual decrease in breathing follows and the breathing can stop temporarily. The breathing cycle can take between 30 seconds and 2 minutes to complete. We observe Cheyne–Stokes respiration in people with congestive heart failure, brain injury, those sleeping at high altitudes and patients who are dying.

In your assessment of respiration, breathing sounds are equally important. Listening to the sounds of breathing in (inspiration) and breathing out (expiration), we can identify respiratory complications. For example, if we hear crackles (high-pitched rustles) at the end of expiration, this may indicate **pulmonary oedema**. If we hear crackles during both inspiration and expiration, this may be an indication of pneumonia (Adam and Osborne 1997).

A further important aspect of respiration is effort to breathe. Effort to breathe is dependent on rate, depth and airway resistance and those with asthma are a typical example of patients who may use the accessory muscles to assist with breathing. During the process, a patient's breathing may be shallow and rapid due to an increase in airway resistance we associate with bronchospasm. The patient may lift the shoulders and use external intercostal muscles during inspiration.

Taking respirations

The procedure

1. *As with any clinical procedure, you need to wash your hands and put on clean gloves and, if necessary, put on a disposable apron.*
2. *Obtain informed consent from the patient and explain the procedure. It is important you allow the patient to ask questions. You should ask your patient if he/she understands the procedure*

continued . . .

before you start. At this time, observe for the following: ability to speak without breathlessness, restlessness, confusion, sweating, or cool, clammy skin, overall skin colour and signs of cyanosis or if the patient's position is constricting the breathing.

3. *Count the respirations over 30 or 60 seconds, depending on the breathing rate.*
4. *Simultaneously, or if you prefer, after counting the respiratory rate, assess rhythm and depth.*
5. *Check the patient's breath sounds using a stethoscope; ensure you assess all lung fields.*
6. *Document the results as soon as possible.*
7. *If there are any changes to the patient's normal respiration, seek assistance and document the changes.*
8. *If unsure at any stage during the assessment, seek guidance from a more experienced member of staff.*

The next important clinical assessment we need to discuss is taking blood pressure.

Blood pressure

Case study

Robert is a 57-year-old man who is the Chief Executive Officer of a successful company. He suffers from bipolar affective disorder and regularly takes mood stabilisers. He has not experienced clinical depressive symptoms for more than 3 years. He plays golf every now and again but, generally, he does not exercise much. His BP is 150/114 mmHg and, at 1.87 m (6 foot 2 inches), he weighs 110 kg (17 stones 4 lb) and his cholesterol level is very high.

BP is the pressure that circulating blood exerts against the walls of blood vessels (Figure 2.3). In other words, it is how strongly the circulating blood presses against the walls of the arteries during the pumping action of the heart. BP does not stay the same; it changes to meet your body's needs. It is one of the most important vital signs, as high or low BP can be an indication of health problems. The case of Robert seems to indicate that something is wrong with homeostasis. Before we discuss the association between BP and health, we need to discuss the mechanisms underlying BP.

When the left ventricle of the heart contracts, it creates pressure that pushes blood into the aorta. Moving blood in the aorta creates pressure against the wall of the aorta, which we call **systolic pressure**. In BP reading, it is usually the top figure. For example, Robert's systolic BP is 150 mmHg. After contraction, the ventricles relax and go into a short rest before contracting again. During ventricular relaxation, the blood exerts a much lower pressure on the wall of the aorta. We call this **diastolic blood pressure** and it is the bottom figure of any BP reading. In Robert's

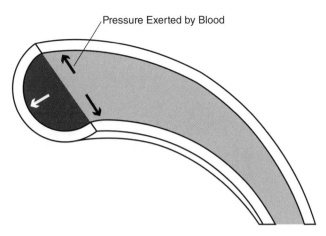

Figure 2.3: Blood pressure

case, the diastolic pressure is 114 mmHg. We call the difference between the systolic and diastolic pressure **pulse pressure**. For example, Robert's pulse pressure is (150–114) = 36. Before you move to the next section, please complete the activity below.

Activity 2.3	*Evidence-based practice and research*

Alone or in a group, can you identify which mental health problems directly affect BP?

As discussed earlier, the circulation of the blood is mainly due to differences in BP from one location to the other. BP in the aorta is higher than the peripherals like the arms, therefore blood flows from the high-pressure aorta to low-pressure arms. In general, average BP decreases as the circulating blood moves away from the heart through arteries, capillaries and veins. The average BP for a 'normal healthy adult' is 120/80 mmHg. It rises steadily throughout childhood, so that in a young adult it might be 120/80 mmHg but as we get older, BP continues to rise. A rule of thumb is that normal systolic pressure is age in years + 100. BP is lower in women in late pregnancy and during sleep. Several factors are responsible for variations in BP and these include age, gender, ethnicity, weight, exercise, stress, emotions and diurnal rhythm. We will briefly discuss each of these factors.

In general, BP tends to rise with increasing age in both males and females after puberty. Before puberty, however, no discernible BP difference exists between males and females. After puberty, males tend to show higher BP readings than females.

After menopause, BP is higher in females than in male counterparts. Another important determinant of BP is ethnicity. There is established evidence suggesting that those of darker skin ethnicity, such as African Caribbean and Asians in the UK and African Americans and Hispanics in the USA, are prone to higher BP (Taylor *et al.* 2012) and we will return to this theme in more detail in Chapter 4.

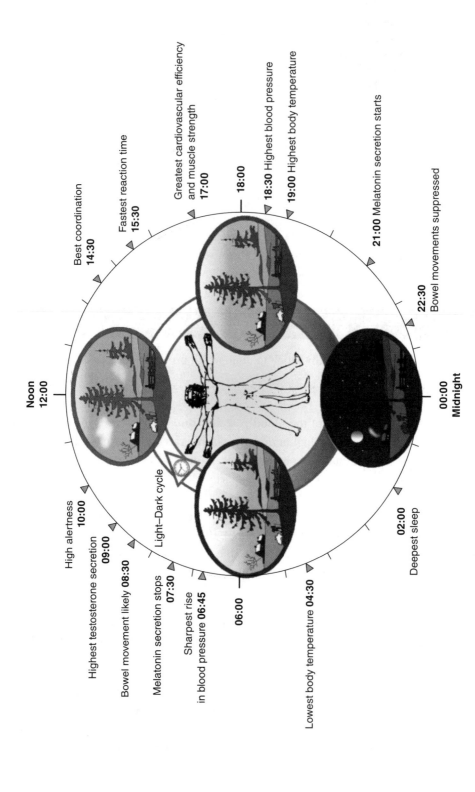

Figure 2.4: The 24-hour biological clock. (Reproduced from Smolensky M, Lamberg L (2000) The Body Clock Guide to Better Health. New York: Henry Holt, with permission)

BP is generally higher in those who are obese and/or those who do not exercise.

The level of stress and emotions affect BP. During periods of fear, anger and pain, BP briefly rises and is relatively low in periods of calm. Equally, if an individual is experiencing stressful life events, it is more than likely s/he will experience high BP.

BP naturally varies during the day (diurnal rhythm). A daily cycle sees BP rise to a peak in the late afternoon or early evening and fall to its lowest during the early hours of the morning, as Figure 2.4 shows.

BP increases with an increase in the volume of blood that the heart pumps per minute, which is cardiac output. The average resting cardiac output for a healthy adult male is approximately 5.6 L/min and that of a healthy female is about 4.9 L/min. Factors that generally increase cardiac output are posture, an increase in sympathetic nervous system activity and a decrease in parasympathetic nervous system activity. Conversely, factors that reduce cardiac output are hypertension, **cardiac myopathy** and heart failure.

Another important factor that determines BP is peripheral vascular resistance (PVR). PVR, also known as systemic vascular resistance, is the opposition to blood flow through the arteries. This resistance occurs when the peripherals of the blood vessels become smaller or they constrict. In this case, the blood requires greater pressure to push it through the constricted vessel (vasoconstriction). Several factors cause vasoconstriction, an important one being tobacco smoking. During smoking, the nicotine in tobacco increases the constriction of blood vessels, therefore increasing PVR. An increase in PVR, as noted earlier, leads to high BP.

Another factor that increases PVR is viscosity of the blood. At its most succinct definition, viscosity is the internal property of a fluid to resist flow. Ordinarily, the less viscous a fluid is, the less resistance to flow it offers, and vice versa. Blood is generally more viscous than water and therefore is more resistant to flow than water in a similar-sized vessel. Put differently, we need more pressure to move blood than to move an equal amount of water moving in a similar-diameter vessel. Before you go any further, please take part in the activity below.

Activity 2.4   *Critical thinking*

Can you suggest a type of medication that changes the viscosity of blood and therefore the BP?

The elasticity of the blood vessel plays a part in the BP level. The more stiff and rigid the blood vessel is, the more pressure that is needed to push through the blood. There are factors that reduce PVR and these are vasodilators, neurochemicals like serotonin, certain types of hormones like relaxin and cholinergic stimulants.

Activity 2.5   *Critical thinking*

Can you think of a vascular illness where the blood vessels harden and are rigid? What is the characteristic of this illness?

Measurement of blood pressure

We traditionally measure BP using a mercury sphygmomanometer, introduced by Riva-Rocci in 1896 and modified by Korotkoff in 1905. This method has served us well over the past 100 years. However, due to technological advances and the banning of environmentally harmful substances such as mercury, the traditional sphygmomanometer is increasingly becoming obsolete. In clinical practice, new approaches to BP measurement that incorporate reliable, automated techniques of measurement have opened new possibilities. Such possibilities include ambulatory (walking) techniques that record BP over 24 hours while the person goes about daily activities. These new developments have reconfigured future BP measurement. Whatever techniques you use, be mindful of important considerations that may lead to inaccurate readings.

You can obtain inaccurate readings through failure to use the proper technique and an inaccurate reading can lead to the wrong diagnosis. This may result in unnecessary or inappropriate treatment and follow-up. So you should not forget the importance of accurate technique in BP measurement. Assessment of nurses' BP reading technique quite often reveals a surprising degree of inaccuracy. To minimise the chances of an inaccurate reading, you should follow the procedure below.

Procedure for measuring blood pressure

1. *As with all nursing procedures, you should observe infection control procedures by ensuring that you wear protective clothing, including gloves and a disposable apron. You need to explain the procedure to the patient and answer any questions the patient may have. In particular, you should warn the patient of the minor discomfort caused by inflation and deflation of the cuff and inform the patient that you may repeat the measurement several times.*
2. *After obtaining consent, you should ensure that the patient is in a warm and comfortable environment that ensures privacy. You should ask the patient to remove tight or restrictive clothing from the arm to which you will apply the cuff. Next, you should mark the position of **maximal pulsation** of the brachial artery in the arm, just above the **antecubital fossa**. Apply the cuff to the upper arm with the lower edge of the cuff about 2–3 cm above the marked point of the antecubital fossa (Figure 2.5). You should fit the cuff firmly and comfortably.*
3. *Before inflating the cuff, you should ensure that the arm is horizontal and supported at the level of the mid-sternum. If the arm hangs below heart level this leads to an overestimation of BP by about 10 mmHg. Conversely, raising the arm above heart level leads to underestimation of BP.*

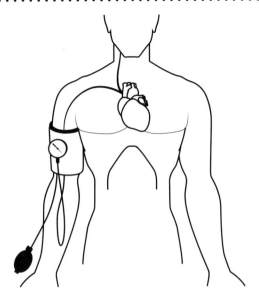

Figure 2.5: Measurement of blood pressure

4. *If you are using a mercury sphygmomanometer, you must ensure the mercury column is vertical, at eye level, and not more than 90 cm from you. Generally, most BP procedure books recommend manometers mounted on a stand, as they are mobile and easy to adjust for height.*
5. *You can estimate the systolic pressure before you use the stethoscope by palpating the brachial artery pulse and inflating the cuff until the pulsation disappears. The point of disappearance represents the systolic pressure. This measure is especially useful in patients in whom **auscultatory gap** may be difficult to judge accurately, for example, pregnant women, patients in shock or those taking exercise.*
6. *Place the stethoscope gently over the artery at the point of maximal pulsation. You must not press too firmly or touch the cuff as this may result in diastolic pressure underestimation. Continue raising the pressure by inflating the bladder to 30 mmHg above the systolic BP, as estimated by palpation.*
7. *Reduce the pressure at a rate of 2–3 mmHg/s: the first appearance of faint, repetitive, clear tapping sounds that gradually increase in intensity for at least two consecutive beats is the systolic BP. The point at which all sounds finally disappear completely is the diastolic pressure.*

Automated blood pressure devices

Most automated devices work on one of three principles: the detection of **Korotkoff sounds** by a microphone or the detection of arterial blood flow by ultrasound or oscillometry. Until recently, automated devices depended on Korotkoff sound detection using an electronic microphone shielded from extraneous noise in the pressure cuff; it then records BP on a print-out or indicates it on a digital display. Because the microphones are sensitive to movement and friction, it is difficult to get accurate readings from electronic microphone-based devices. Manufacturers are turning therefore to oscillometric detection of BP, in which cuff placement is not critical.

As with all equipment, you should seek advice from the manufacturer for evidence of validation of the equipment.

Electrocardiogram

In simple terms, an ECG is a test that measures the electrical activity of the heart muscle at skin level; Willem Einthoven (1860–1927) pioneered this test. An ECG test continues to be a critical component of the evaluation of patients with cardiac symptoms. It is a fast, efficient and non-invasive method of diagnosing abnormal rhythms of the heart which we can conduct in most places (Braunwald 1997). In mental health nursing, ECGs are now in frequent use to monitor heart function and this is particularly so for those patients taking antipsychotics such as olanzapine, clozapine or tricyclic antidepressants (Mutsatsa 2011).

The ECG machine detects and amplifies minute electrical changes on the skin that result from depolarisation of the heart muscle during each heart beat, as shown in Figure 2.6.

When the heart is at rest, each heart muscle cell has a negative charge across its cell membrane, called the membrane potential. During depolarisation of the heart muscle cell, calcium (Ca^+) and sodium (Na^+) ions enter the cell, causing a less negative charge inside the cell, activating the mechanisms in the cell that cause it to contract. This process of depolarisation starts in the sino-atrial node (see Chapter 4) and spreads throughout the atrium. From the atrium, depolarisation passes through the atrioventricular node before it spreads all over the ventricles via the interventricular septum. The ECG detects these events as tiny rises and falls in the voltage,

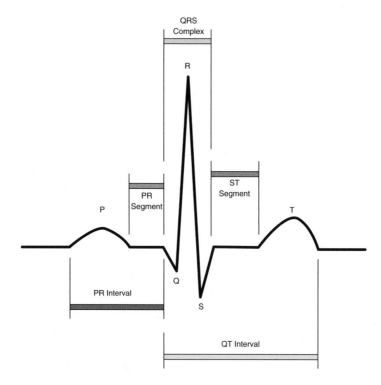

Figure 2.6: Changes in electrical activity of the heart

ECG section	Explanation
PR interval	This is the time from the start of the P wave to the start of the QRS complex. It reflects conduction through the atrioventricular node
PQ interval or PR segment	This is the flat segment where we do not detect variation in cell voltage (isoelectric). It lies between the end of the P wave and the start of the QRS complex. Abnormalities in this segment could be an indication of pericarditis or atrial ischaemia
QRS complex	This section corresponds to the depolarisation of the right and left ventricles of the heart. In healthy adults, it normally lasts 0.06–0.10 seconds. It is usually shorter during physical activity and in children
The QT interval	The QT interval is the time from the start of the Q wave to the end of the T wave. It represents the time taken for ventricular depolarisation and repolarisation. The QT interval is inversely proportional to heart rate. The QT shortens at faster heart rates and is longer at slower heart rates
ST segment	This is the flat section where the ECG does not detect any voltage between the end of the S wave and the beginning of the T wave. It represents the interval between ventricular depolarisation and repolarisation. ST-segment abnormality could be an indication of myocardial ischaemia or myocardial infarction
P wave	This is the first positive deflection on the ECG that represents atrial depolarisation
T wave	This is the positive deflection after each QRS complex and it represents the repolarisation of the ventricles

Table 2.1: Sections of the electrocardiogram (ECG) waves

as Figure 2.6 illustrates. Table 2.1 explains each particular section of the ECG, as shown in Figure 2.6, and its implication.

Machine preparation

Before you use the ECG machine, you should ensure the machine is clean and is in a usable state. Preferably, you should clean it with alcohol and gauze to minimise the chances of cross-infection. Additionally, you should check if the machine has sufficient ECG paper for recording results. Connect the power cord to a wall outlet; some ECG machines use a back-up built-in battery unit for situations where mains power is not accessible.

Patient preparation

You should let the patient know your intentions and agree a time for ECG recording. Explain the procedure in a way that the patient understands without being patronising and ensure privacy for the occasion. You need to reassure the patient that there is no danger or pain involved. Encourage the patient to ask questions and answer any questions honestly.

You should ask the patient to remove clothing above the waist and wear a cloth gown. At this stage, you should be sensitive to the privacy needs of the patient relating to gender and culture. Ensure the patient is comfortable lying down on the examination table and the legs, arms and chest area are exposed. If necessary, you should shave the electrode areas before cleaning the exposed skin with alcohol to remove oil, sweat or scaly skin for proper electrode adhesion. At all times follow correct infection control precautions according to local policy.

Application of limb sensors

Attach the sensors on a smooth area of the upper arms and lower legs at the positions shown in Figure 2.7.

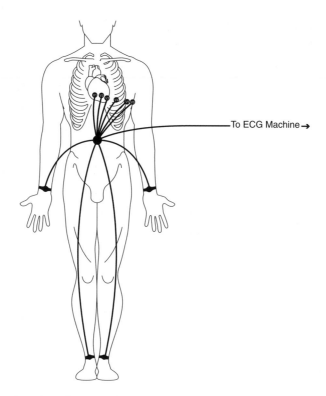

To ECG Machine →

Figure 2.7: Application sites of sensors

Chest sensor applications

After applying the limb sensors, attach the six chest sensors at the positions shown in Figure 2.7 as follows:

- Attach V1 to the fourth intercostal space at the right border of the sternum.
- Attach V2 to the fourth intercostal space at the left border of the sternum.

- Attach V3 to midway between position V2 and position V4.

- Attach V4 at the mid-clavicular line in the fifth intercostal space.

- Attach V5 at the anterior axillary line on the same horizontal level as V4.

- Attach V6 at the mid-axillary line on the same horizontal level as V4 and V5.

Recording the ECG

After switching the ECG machine on, you should wait 10 seconds for it to stabilise.

Press the record button and print the results, which you should send to a doctor or specialist for interpretation.

We now turn our attention to peak flow – another important assessment in physical health.

Peak flow

Case study

Susan is 32 years old and suffers from obsessive compulsive disorder and has had asthma since she was 7 years old. As part of her treatment, she inhales corticosteroids and bronchodilators. However, one summer morning, she was admitted to hospital with an acute asthma exacerbation. She had increased wheeze, cough, yellow sputum and chest tightness. Susan's peak flow was 250 L/min (normal range at her age is 380–518 L/min) and she was given hydrocortisone and aminophylline intravenously. After a week of treatment in hospital, Susan was discharged with her lowest peak flow reading at 350 L/min and highest at 450 L/min.

As part of the physical health assessment, you will be required to measure the rate of expiration of your patient. This is particularly important in patients like Susan who have respiratory problems such as asthma. Peak expiratory flow (PEF) or simply peak flow is the measurement of the highest rate at which the lungs can expel air from the lungs through an open mouth. We use it to indicate any restriction to the airway and it is a useful assessment for patients with asthma or other respiratory symptoms. We measure PEF using a small device which we hold in the hand and it measures the flow of air through the bronchi and thus the extent of obstruction in the airways.

When a patient with respiratory problems is well, peak flow is normally high; conversely, peak flows are low when the patient is unwell (see Figure 2.8 for normal values). For example, when Susan was having an asthma attack, her peak flow was 250 L/min, suggesting very low levels of oxygen supply to the body. Weak peak flow can indicate several factors, including poor technique of use of the PEF meter, poor management of the respiratory condition or poor treatment adherence by the patient. By recording peak flow, we can determine lung functionality and, in the case of asthma, severity of symptoms and treatment options. In Susan's case, the treatment team were able to make the decision to discharge her when her flow reading was consistently above 350 L/min.

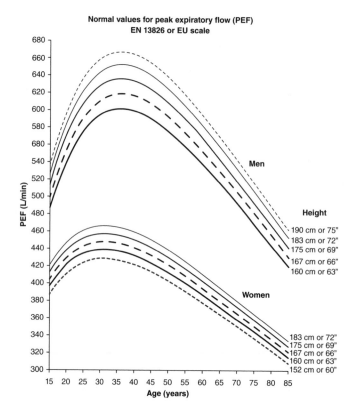

Figure 2.8: Normal peak flows for men and women

You will need to train patients on the correct use of the PEF meter to obtain accurate readings. A normal PEF value depends on a patient's gender, age and height (Figure 2.8). In people suffering from asthma or obstructive lung disorders, PEF values are very low.

We obtain peak flow measurement using a spirometer. This instrument has a mouthpiece that measures the amount and rate of air we breathe in or out of the lungs. We usually perform spirometry at a health clinic, GP practice or a hospital. At times, we measure peak flow using a peak flow meter (PFM), a portable, hand-held device. A PFM is small and light enough to use almost anywhere. Both a spirometer and PFM device take the measurement as an individual forcefully blows into the mouthpiece. There are several types of PFMs available. However, it is important that you consistently use the same type of PFM, as the PEF can vary among different brands and types of meters. Before you read the procedures, please take part in the next activity.

Activity 2.6   *Critical thinking*

Incorporating your knowledge of previous sections of this chapter, would you expect Susan's respiration rate and pulse rate to be increased or decreased? Why?

Procedure for peak flow measurement

1. *As with all clinical procedures, you should observe local infection control guidelines.*
2. *You need to explain the procedure to the patient and obtain informed consent. Encourage the patient to ask questions if he/she wants and answer questions honestly. Ensure privacy during the process.*
3. *Ask the patient to stand and blow into the meter as hard as he/she is able to. Ask the patient to repeat the procedure a couple more times and record only the highest reading of the three.*
4. *Dispose of the used mouthpiece.*
5. *If the readings you obtain are abnormal, communicate this finding to the team.*

Oximeter oxygen rate

The measurement of saturated oxygen levels (SpO_2) is important because our body requires a continuous supply of oxygen for cellular activity to take place. Assessing your patient's need for oxygen is critical; no human life thrives without oxygen.

Inadequate oxygen supply will result in cell death that can lead to a host of complications, including delirium, cardiac ischaemia and malfunctioning of vital organs. Continued lack of oxygen in the body will result in death.

We measure the oxygen saturation rate of an individual using an instrument we call an oximeter. Pulse oximetry is a simple non-invasive method of monitoring the percentage of oxygen saturation in the blood. The instrument (oximeter) consists of a probe that we attach to the patient's finger or earlobe and it links to a computerised unit which displays the percentage of blood saturated with oxygen, pulse beat and heart rate. One key advantage of an oximeter is that it can detect low levels of oxygen saturation (hypoxia) before the patient becomes clinically cyanosed. Cyanosis is the appearance of a bluish discoloration of the skin, fingernails and mucous membranes caused by a deficiency of oxygen in the blood. A healthy individual at sea level usually shows oxygen saturation values between 96% and 99%. An oxygen saturation level of below 90% usually indicates a reduction of oxygen supply to body tissues below physiological levels (hypoxia). An oximeter works by emitting red light (600–750 nm wavelength) and infrared light (850–1000 nm wavelength). The light is partly absorbed by haemoglobin in the blood and the amount of light absorbed differs depending on whether the blood is saturated with oxygen (oxygenated) or not. Oxygenated blood absorbs more infrared light and allows more red light to pass through. Conversely, deoxygenated blood absorbs more red light and allows more infrared light to pass through it.

Pulse oximetry is a particularly easy and non-invasive method of measuring blood SpO_2 levels. Its simplicity of use allows for the provision of continuous and immediate oxygen saturation values and this is particularly important in emergencies and in patients with respiratory or cardiac problems. However, it has limitations; oxygen saturation is only one factor in oxygenation of the tissues. In anaemia, for example, it is possible to have high oxygen saturation readings even if inadequate amounts of oxygen reach the tissues. In addition, during carbon monoxide exposure, haemoglobin prefers carbon monoxide to oxygen molecules. Because blood with carbon monoxide is also bright red, this can lead to significant overestimation of oxygen saturation when using pulse oximeters.

Procedure for pulse oximetry

1. *Start by explaining to your patient that you need to take an oxygen saturation reading and obtain consent. You should ensure your patient understands the procedure and answer any questions s/he might have.*
2. *Next, you should ensure that the patient is comfortable and warm enough, particularly if you are continuously monitoring the patient. Apart from patient comfort, shivering can interfere with the pulse oximeter reading.*
3. *Before using the probe and equipment, you should ensure it is clean to minimise the risk of cross-infection.*
4. *Wash your hands with soap and water or use alcohol gel to decontaminate and minimise the risk of cross-infection.*
5. *Select a suitable area for the probe (usually fingertip), or you can use other sites like earlobes, bridge of nose or toes.*
6. *Place the probe as directed by the manufacturer's instructions, assessing any barriers such as nail varnish, nicotine staining or dirt. This is because intravenous dyes, poor perfusion and skin pigmentation will affect pulse oximeter readings.*
7. *Note and record the reading from the oximeter and then remove the probe and ensure the patient is comfortable.*

Now we will look at another assessment that is equally important – the measurement of blood sugar levels.

Blood sugar levels

Case study

Peter is a 50-year-old male of African Caribbean origin who has suffered from schizophrenia for the last 25 years. He has had several admissions to hospital but his condition is currently stable. He has been taking olanzapine medication for the past 10 years and 2 years ago, he was diagnosed with type 2 diabetes. He takes his blood sugar levels before meals using a glucometer. His blood sugar levels tend to average 2.5 mmol/L before meals and 20 mmol/L after meals.

Glucose is a simple sugar that is a major source of energy for most cells of the body, including those in the brain, heart, liver and other vital organs. We express the concentration of blood glucose level in mmol/L. As part of homeostasis, the body tightly regulates blood glucose levels and the average for a healthy person fluctuates between 4 and 6 mmol/L before a meal. Blood sugar level is normally lowest in the morning, before breakfast (4–6 mmol/L) and rises after meals (8–10 mmol/L). Blood glucose concentrations that fall outside the range of 4–10 mmol/L give rise to troubling conditions, including hypoglycaemia, as with Peter's blood glucose level before and after meals. If the blood glucose level is above 10 mmol/L, we call this state hyper-glycaemic. Peter's blood sugar levels of 20 mmol/L after meals adequately describe the condition. We will discuss this condition in more detail in Chapter 5. For now, we need to look at how we monitor blood glucose levels. Like Peter, we monitor blood glucose using a glucometer and there are several types of instruments available commercially. Despite their differences, you should adopt a similar procedure.

Blood glucose testing procedure

1. *Prepare by having to hand: alcohol preparation pad, finger-lancing device, blood glucose testing meter (there are several types, such as Accu-Chek Advantage, LifeScan, UltraOne), blood testing strips, tissue or cotton balls, spot bandage, pair of gloves. Next, explain the procedure to the patient, answer any questions s/he might have and obtain informed consent.*
2. *You should put gloves on, clean the area you want to lance with an alcohol swab and ensure the test site is dry before lancing, as moisture (water or alcohol) that remains on the skin may alter the test results.*
3. *Check the glucose testing strip expiry dates and that it is in good working order before you insert the strip into the electronic meter according to the manufacturer's instructions.*
4. *Prepare the lancing device according to the manufacturer's instructions.*
5. *You should then select a site: if a finger, then the top side of the fingertip is most appropriate. Before you lance the site, you should ask the patient to hang the arm below the level of the heart for 30 seconds to increase blood flow.*
6. *Puncture the site with the lancing device and note that the tops of the fingertips may be more sensitive for the patient. If this is the case, then you should use other sites such as the forearm.*
7. *You should gently squeeze the finger in a downward motion to obtain a large enough drop of blood to cover the test strip.*
8. *Place the blood on the testing strip and complete according to manufacturer's instructions. Compress lanced area with tissue or cotton ball until bleeding stops or apply spot bandage.*
9. *Dispose of test strip and tissue or cotton ball in a lined wastebasket and dispose of the lancing device (if it's a disposable type) in a sharps container.*
10. *Remove and dispose of gloves and wash your hands.*
11. *Ensure that your patient is all right and offer reassurance if necessary.*

Body mass index

The BMI is a proxy measure of human body fat pioneered by the Belgian mathematician Quetelet (1796–1874). The BMI bases an individual's body fat on weight and height and does not actually measure the percentage of an individual's fat (Keys *et al.* 1972). We define BMI as the individual's body mass divided by the square of the individual's height (Figure 2.9). Thus:

BMI = mass (kg) ÷ height (metres²)

Because of its simplicity, BMI is popular, but it is important to know that its use as a true measure of a person's fat content is controversial. Many professionals, including nurses, have come to rely on its supposed objective numerical authority to make authoritative diagnosis but, in truth, that was never the intended purpose of BMI (WHO 1995). Instead, we should use it as a simple means of classifying physically inactive (sedentary) populations, with an average body composition. Another common use of the BMI is to assess how much an individual's body weight departs from what is 'normal or desirable' for a person of his or her height. We can partly explain excess weight or underweight by body fat (adipose tissue), but other factors such as muscularity also significantly affect BMI. It generally overestimates body fat in those with more lean body mass, such as athletes, and underestimates excess adiposity on those with less lean body mass.

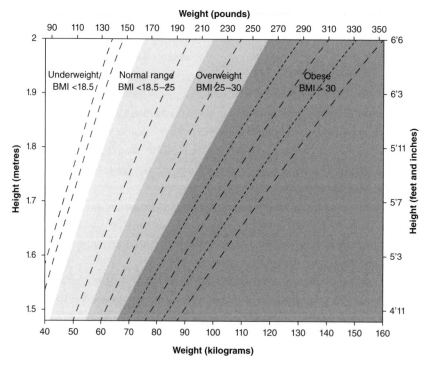

Figure 2.9: The relationship between weight, height and body mass index (BMI)

The World Health Organization (WHO) has devised an international classification of adult underweight, overweight and obesity according to BMI (Table 2.2).

Classification	BMI (kg/m²)	
	Principal cut-off points	**Additional cut-off points**
Underweight	**<18.50**	**<18.50**
Severe thinness	<16.00	<16.00
Moderate thinness	16.00–16.99	16.00–16.99
Mild thinness	17.00–18.49	17.00–18.49
Normal range	**18.50–24.99**	**18.50–22.99**
		23.00–24.99
Overweight	**≥25.00**	**≥25.00**
Pre-obese	25.00–29.99	25.00–27.49
		27.50–29.99
Obese	**≥30.00**	**≥30.00**
Obese class I	30.00–34.99	30.00–32.49
		32.50–34.99
Obese class II	35.00–39.99	35.00–37.49
		37.50–39.99
Obese class III	≥40.00	≥40.00

Table 2.2: International classification of adult underweight, overweight and obesity according to body mass index (BMI)

Adapted from World Health Organization (2004).

An additional problem of BMI usage is quantifying and standardising BMI to different populations and ethnic groups. This is problematic because such an approach assumes that these groups have similar risks of morbidity and mortality at similar levels of BMI, but there is no evidence to suggest that this assumption is valid (de Onis and Habicht 1996). Indeed, limited evidence suggesting that people of Chinese origin have a higher prevalence of disease at lower BMI levels than Caucasians prompted the WHO to recommend that overweight status for Orientals be based on a BMI of 23.0–24.9 (International Diabetes Institute 2000). This is because people of Chinese origin have smaller frames than Caucasians, and therefore higher levels of body fat at similar BMIs (Deurenberg *et al.* 1999; Nazare *et al.* 2012).

To overcome the problems posed by BMI, we now recommend waist circumference and waist–hip ratio as a more accurate measure. A recent study followed up 60,000 participants for up to 13 years and found that waist–hip ratio is a better predictor of ischaemic heart disease mortality than BMI (Morkedal *et al.* 2011).

Waist circumference and waist–hip ratio

The WHO Expert Consultation on Obesity recognised the importance of waist–hip ratio (referred to as abdominal, central or visceral obesity) (WHO 2008b). Abdominal body mass is important and can vary considerably within a narrow range of BMI and, as we previously discussed, there is evidence to suggest it is a more accurate predictor of cardiovascular disease (de Hert *et al.* 2007). An early longitudinal study that followed up middle-aged men for 12 years strongly supports this approach. The study showed abdominal obesity (measured as waist–hip ratio) was associated with an increased risk of myocardial infarction, stroke and premature death, whereas these diseases were not associated with measures of generalised obesity, such as BMI (Larsson *et al.* 1984). Recent studies also support the use of waist–hip ratio (Morkedal *et al.* 2011).

We measure waist circumference at the midpoint between the lower margin of the least palpable rib and the top of the iliac crest, using a stretch-resistant tape (WHO 2011c). We measure hip circumference around the widest portion of the buttocks, with the tape parallel to the floor. For both measurements, you should ensure the patient is standing with feet close together, arms at the side and body weight evenly distributed, and wearing little clothing. Encourage the patient to relax and take the measurement at the end of normal expiration. Repeat each measurement twice; if the measurements are within 1 cm of one another, then calculate the average.

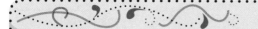

Chapter summary

In this chapter, we discussed that homeostasis is the ability or tendency of an organism or cell to maintain internal equilibrium by adjusting its physiological processes. From time to time, the body fails to maintain a stable internal environment, and this leads to accumulation of toxins and destruction of cell and tissues, which are threats to life. This is particularly so as our body ages, and as a result, we need to monitor indicators of homeostasis. Such indicators typically involve the monitoring of BP, pulse, respiration, temperature, ECG, blood glucose and BMI, among others. With particular reference to BMI, it is a less accurate approximate of body fat content than other measures and therefore we should use it sparingly. Correct monitoring of proxies of homeostasis assist us in providing the correct care to our patients.

Activities: brief outline answers

Activity 2.1

Your list may have included hypoglycaemia, diabetes, hypertension, hypotension, cardiac arrhythmia, cancer, asthma and respiratory diseases.

Activity 2.2

People with dementia, unconscious, restless, young children, paranoid breathing difficulties or dental problems, hypothermia, heat stroke.

Activity 2.3

Anxiety, depression.

Activity 2.4

Anticoagulants.

Activity 2.5

Arteriosclerosis, characterised by high BP.

Activity 2.6

Both should be increased: to compensate for lack of oxygen in the body due the asthma attack, the heart will increase its pumping rate, although it will be weaker. This increases the pulse and respiration rate.

Further reading

Blows WT (2012) *The Biological Basis of Clinical Observations*, 2nd edn. London: Routledge.

This is a useful book that covers the biological mechanism of clinical observation in more depth.

Useful websites

http://www.medicine.mcgill.ca/physio/vlab/cardio/ECGbasics.htm
http://publications.nice.org.uk/hypertension-cg127

These National Institute for Health and Care Excellence guidelines have more information on hypertension and its management.

http://www.ecglibrary.com/ecghome.html

This website has very good diagrams and an accessible explanation of the heart and ECG.

Chapter 3
Physical health promotion, communication and the therapeutic alliance

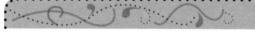

Introduction

Case study

Tina is a 37-year-old woman who has suffered from anxiety since she was 18 years old. She smokes 15 cigarettes and drinks half a bottle of wine a day. She has no known physical health problems but her average blood pressure from several readings over the last 4 months is 190/102 mmHg. Other physical findings are unremarkable, including electrolytes, full blood count, lipids, glucose and uric acid tests, which were normal. Despite the advice by the community nurse to take more exercise and restrict her dietary salt intake, she has not changed her lifestyle.

As a nurse, how would you promote Tina's health? To be able to understand health promotion, we need to understand the concept of health. However, a universal definition of health is elusive, as it is one of those abstract words like love or beauty that mean different things to different people. We might say that Tina is not healthy, but it is possible to say that she is healthy and Tina herself would probably say she is. One of the most enduring debates is whether 'health' means being well, or not being ill. In 2006, the World Health Organization (WHO) defined health as *a state of complete physical, mental and social well-being and not merely the absence of disease or infirmity* (Sampson *et al.* 2006). This definition allows people to see health in a variety of ways. It is therefore important for you to acknowledge the multidimensional and holistic nature of health and its central importance in people's lives.

The way people view their health informs and shapes how they respond to health threats. For example, Tina does not seem to perceive any health threats (we will cover this in later sections) so is not making any changes. In turn, people's view of their health status informs your health promotion strategy. In Tina's case, she shows no concern for her health and, therefore, the health promotion strategy you should employ should take account of this reality.

This chapter will explore the concept of health and health promotion models that lie behind nursing intervention strategies. We will discuss the concepts of health promotion, the therapeutic alliance and ways of motivating people to adopt behaviours that promote health.

First, we discuss the importance of health promotion in mental health.

Health promotion

According to the WHO, health promotion is *the process of enabling people to increase control over, and to improve, their health in order for them to reach a state of complete physical, mental and social well-being* (WHO 2014a). In their assertion, the WHO sees health as a resource for everyday life, not the reason for living. This positive concept of health emphasises physical capacities and social and personal resources.

Apart from health as a major resource for social, economic and personal development, it is also an important dimension of quality of life (WHO 2009). It moves beyond a focus on individual behaviour towards a wide range of social and environmental intervention. For example, in Tina's case, we see that aspects of her lifestyle, such as drinking and smoking, compromise her health. According to the contemporary view, health promotion in Tina's case aims to make conditions favourable for her to choose a healthier lifestyle. These should include addressing those factors that make her unable or unwilling to have a healthier lifestyle, such as access to information, life skills and opportunities for making healthy choices. People cannot achieve their fullest health potential unless they are able to take control of those things which determine their health. Therefore, health promotion is not just the responsibility of the individual; health promotion must focus on the wider influences on health, including the social determinants of health.

As nurses, we can structure health promotion in people with mental health problems as a combination of health education, health protection and health policy. We can define health education as any planned activity that we design to produce health- or illness-related learning. Health protection is concerned with developing and implementing legislation, policies and programmes to protect the public from environmental hazards (air quality, drinking water, food safety, diseases carried by mammals and insects). In the UK, the Health Protection Agency is one such organisation that is responsible for health protection. We can define the third aspect of health promotion (health policy) as the decisions, plans and actions that governments take to hasten particular healthcare priorities within a society. For example, current government policy is to make it easier for those who want to give up smoking by offering them support by empowering them. Nevertheless, before we discuss the concept of empowerment in more detail, please take part in the activity below.

Activity 3.1   *Critical thinking*

Read again the case study of Tina. As she is not complaining of any symptoms of a physical disease, can we describe her as healthy?

There are outline answers to all the activities at the end of the chapter.

Empowerment

> ### Case study
>
> *Kofi is a 24-year-old young man who has recently recovered from an episode of bipolar disorder. He lives alone in a one-bedroomed flat. He has concerns about his ever-increasing weight and recently, he saw a documentary on TV suggesting that eating fruit and vegetables can help to reduce weight. He would like to buy more fruit and vegetables but his weekly income is not sufficient. He therefore feels powerless to lose weight.*

Many people with mental health problems feel powerless, like Kofi, for a variety of reasons, as we will see later. In order to understand powerlessness we first need to grasp the concept of power. We define power simply as the ability to influence the behaviour of people. When we apply power legitimately, we call this authority, but if we apply it illegitimately, we call this coercion.

In contrast to power, powerlessness is the perception that one's own action will not significantly affect an outcome or a perceived lack of control over a current situation or immediate happening. For example, Kofi may feel that whatever he does in relation to his weight, he is doomed to gain weight and this feeling of powerlessness is pervasive in people with mental health problems. Therefore, we need to empower as many people as possible who have mental health problems. Empowerment is simply taking corrective action towards the lack of control and sense of helplessness that patients develop over many years of interacting with mental health services. We will discuss this concept in later sections but before you read further, please take part in the activity below.

> ### Activity 3.2   *Decision making*
>
> If you were Kofi's nurse, what measures could you take in corroboration with him to empower him to keep to a healthy weight?

In your attempt to promote physical health and well-being in people with mental health problems, you should aim to empower them through the application of health-promoting strategies. Empowerment emerges from a sense of autonomy that arises from knowledge, self-confidence and the availability of meaningful choices. If you apply health promotion theories correctly, this should help to empower patients, and it is these theories we will discuss next.

Health promotion theories

In trying to understand how people react differently to health-related matters, psychologists mostly use models of social cognition theory. These models try to identify the main beliefs, or 'cognitive tenets' that affect the way people deal with the external factors influencing how they behave in health-related matters. Such external factors are both demographic and social. These include age, gender, culture, religion and education.

Theoretical models or frameworks that have wide application are the Health Belief Model (Becker *et al.* 1974), Health Locus of Control (Seeman and Seeman 1983), Protection Motivation Theory (Maddux and Rogers 1983), Theory of Reasoned Action/Planned Behaviour (Ajzen 1991), Self-Efficacy Theory (Bandura 1977b) and Self-Regulation Theory (Leventhal *et al.* 1984). All of these models assume that individuals are rational beings whose health-related behaviour depends upon their understanding of relevant information. The models have all been widely applied to a range of physical illnesses and, overall, they have explained the differences in illness-related behaviours, which makes it easier to intervene by challenging the beliefs held (Connor and Norman 1995). For the purpose of physical health promotion in mental health, we will briefly discuss the Health Belief Model, the Self-Efficacy Theory, Prochaska and DiClemente's Stages of Change Model and the Self-Regulation Model (SRM).

The Health Belief Model

The Health Belief Model was first developed in the 1950s by social psychologists Hochbaum, Rosenstock and Kegels, working in the US Public Health Services. It was developed in response to the failure of a free tuberculosis health screening programme and since then, the Health Belief Model has been adapted to explore a variety of long- and short-term health behaviours, including sexually risky behaviours and the transmission of HIV/AIDS. It attempts to explain and predict health behaviours of people by focusing on their attitudes and beliefs. It considers five main areas that are likely to influence health-seeking behaviour (Mutsatsa 2011). The areas are:

1. how susceptible they feel to disease (specific or non-specific);
2. how serious that disease is likely to be;
3. what benefits, disadvantages and barriers to acting upon those perceptions are likely to exist (for each course of action);
4. how likely the patient is to change;
5. what triggers exist to transform the accumulated concern into an actual action.

To put this more simply, and from a patient's viewpoint:

1. Am I going to get the disease?
2. How bad would it be?
3. How easy would it be to get something done about it? What is it going to cost me?
4. Am I able to make any changes?
5. OK, now I am going to do something about it!

Perceived susceptibility

For a given condition, patients will have a perception of how susceptible they are to developing the illness. Patients may base this perception on experience: they might have a parent or sibling with the disease and therefore convince themselves that they too will get it. Conversely, they may feel that they are somehow not vulnerable to certain diseases. For example, Tina might refuse to give up smoking because she knows a lifelong smoker who has never had any health problems.

Perceived seriousness

Patients differ in how serious they consider various conditions to be, and this interacts with their perception of susceptibility. For instance, a patient may be at low risk of developing bowel cancer, but since s/he perceives it as a very serious condition, s/he may feel motivated to see the doctor about persisting loose stools. Another patient may consider a headache a triviality, feel that seeing the doctor would be a waste of the doctor's time, and therefore possibly fail to have a serious condition diagnosed.

Perception of seriousness can affect not only whether patients present to a healthcare service, but also where they present. If patients feel that coughing up green phlegm is serious, they may consult their doctor, but if they consider it trivial, they may take the problem to a pharmacist. This last point is important because it also interacts with cultural factors and you may want to take part in the activity below before proceeding further.

Activity 3.3 — *Critical thinking*

Kareena is a 37-year-old woman of South Asian origin who suffers from schizophrenia and has recently been diagnosed with type 1 diabetes. She believes that the illness has been caused by a lack of balance between air and space (*vāta*), fire and water (*pitta*) and water and earth (*kapha*). She has sought traditional Hindu methods of healing and refused insulin therapy.

Is Kareena's view of her condition invalid?

Perceived benefits and barriers

Quite often, patients face different options in how to deal with their health concerns. They will often weigh up the potential benefits and drawbacks to each course of action and consider any perceived barriers to health-seeking activity. How patients decide which route to take, and the importance they attach to individual benefits, disadvantages and barriers of health seeking, may differ markedly from person to person.

Self-efficacy

We use the term self-efficacy to describe how people view their own ability to carry out a particular action. We define it as *people's beliefs about their capabilities to exercise control over events that affect their lives* and their *beliefs in their capabilities to mobilise the motivation, cognitive resources, and courses of action needed to exercise control over task demands* (Bandura 1991). Therefore, self-efficacy attributions are concerned *not with the skills one has but with the judgements of what one can do with whatever skills one possesses*. This includes patients' perception of how likely they are to change particular behaviours. For example, a patient may well realise that if he continues to smoke he may well get, and die from, heart disease. The patient may have spoken to the GP about this many times and the GP may offer treatment to stop smoking. However, the patient may feel that he will never be able to stop smoking, so does not think it worth the effort. A perception of low self-efficacy is the barrier to taking action in this case.

Cues to action

Even when patients develop a perception about their health, a trigger turns this into action. From a communication viewpoint, you will want to uncover what triggered a patient to seek healthcare. The possible triggers may be many and different: the media, a relative, an overheard conversation or a reminder letter. Such a prompt may increase patients' perception of their susceptibility to a disease or of its seriousness; it may remind them of the benefits of seeking healthcare. The prompt may increase their motivation to change, or convince them that they may in fact be able to make the necessary changes themselves.

Like all theoretical models, the Health Belief Model has some limitations. For this reason, it has been modified over time and the influence of culture, society (media, etc.) and demographic factors are all important modifiers that should be considered. One other influential model is Bandura's Self-Efficacy Model (Bandura 1977a).

The Self-Efficacy Theory

Since the Self-Efficacy Theory was developed, it has become one of the key theoretical frameworks in most social psychological models. Self-efficacy, as we have seen, refers to the confidence individuals have in their ability to take action and persist in action. For example, in Activity 3.3, Kareena has self-efficacy to overcome symptoms of diabetes. At least four factors influence self-efficacy: direct experience, physiological state, verbal persuasion and vicarious experience, and we will describe these next.

The previous experience of the individual may shape his/her confidence and belief to overcome a particular situation. For example, a retired sportsman may have high confidence and belief in coping with an exercise programme to reduce weight.

In terms of physiological state, people rely partly on information from their physiological state in judging their capabilities. A good example is of someone who is obese and struggles to walk up the stairs without being breathless. The person is likely to have low confidence in coping with an exercise programme because his physiological state is informing him so.

Verbal persuasion may take the form of talking people into believing that they possess the capabilities that enable them to achieve what they seek. At a practical level, you can use various well-recognised attitude change techniques.

The fourth element that influences self-efficacy is vicarious information. This incorporates the view that people judge their capabilities partly by comparing their performance with that of others. In this respect, an individual who might initially have low confidence in taking part in a weight loss programme may feel confident if a friend has successfully taken part.

Overall, self-efficacy is one of the most valuable and practical features of health promotion. It links well with the transtheoretical model of change, which we will discuss next.

The transtheoretical model of change

The transtheoretical model of change was developed to explain how individuals move towards adopting health-enhancing behaviour (Prochaska and DiClemente 1984).

It assesses an individual's readiness to act on a new healthier behaviour and provides processes of change to guide the individual. The individual passes through a series of stages when addressing problematic behaviour (Figure 3.1). This is because behavioural changes are not usually instant but involve several steps, taken over time. These steps are pre-contemplation, contemplation, preparation, taking action and maintenance. We will discuss these next.

Individuals in the *pre-contemplation* stage may not believe that changing behaviour such as stopping smoking is important and may not have any desire to change. At the *contemplation* stage, the person is thinking of changing behaviour but not fully dedicated to changing. Typically, the person is more aware that smoking can be problematic to health. In the *preparation* stage, the person is intending to stop smoking, but may have several barriers preventing him/her from doing so. Individuals who are *taking action* are actively working to stop smoking while those in the *maintenance* stage are doing so on a consistent basis.

In deciding to change a current behaviour, individuals must balance the pros and cons of the change according to their lifestyles and health beliefs (Prochaska and DiClemente 1984). As people move from unawareness of any problem, through contemplating a change, to actually carrying out the action, the pros increase and the cons decrease. Once individuals accomplish

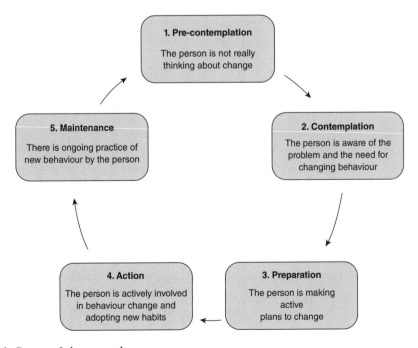

Figure 3.1: Stages of change cycle

Stage of change	Process in operation/explanation	Patient characteristics	Possible intervention
Stage 1 Precontemplation	1. Consciousness raising 2. Social liberation	1. Rebellion 2. Resignation 3. Rationalisation 4. Reluctance	1. Provide choices 2. Build hope 3. Encourage reflection 4. Give information 5. Reinforce progress
Stage 2 Contemplation	1. Consciousness raising 2. Social liberation 3. Emotional arousal 4. Self-evaluation 5. Commitment	1. Open to information 2. Ambivalence	1. Provide information 2. Help to weigh pros and cons 3. Increase self-efficacy 4. Reinforce progress
Stage 3 Preparation	1. Social liberation 2. Emotional arousal 3. Self re-evaluation	Determination	1. Help set goals 2. Provide strategies for change 3. Reinforce progress
Stage 4 Action	1. Social liberation 2. Commitment 3. Reward 4. Environmental control 5. Helping relationships	1. Actively changing 2. Self-evaluation	1. Teach skills and self-management 2. Guide attribution process 3. Reinforce progress
Stage 5 Maintenance	1. Commitment 2. Reward 3. Countering 4. Environmental control 5. Helping relationships	1. At risk/relapse 2. Self-evaluation	1. Teach relapse prevention strategies 2. Encourage continuation 3. Reinforce progress

Table 3.1: Stages of change and associated patient characteristics and possible interventions

the change, self-efficacy or the confidence to overcome difficulties and maintain the new behaviour pattern is important (Julius *et al.* 2009).

You will need to reinforce any progress and encourage the patient during the entire process of change. In the early stages of change, emotional and cognitive factors are important to raise consciousness and increase motivation to take the first step. In the later stages, there is more emphasis on commitment, action and avoiding relapse; defining goals and teaching health-sustaining activities and relapse prevention strategies become more important. We need to gear motivation and supplying relevant information specifically to the patient's stage of readiness to change (Table 3.1).

These stages are not absolute. People may move slowly or rapidly between them, sometimes appearing to miss stages completely, or may remain stuck at one stage. They may hold actions and thoughts relating to more than one stage simultaneously and may move forwards or backwards. However, it is important not to pressurise the patient as this may lead to resistance. In some instances, health promotional theories such as the SRM are more applicable.

Self-Regulatory Model

Case study

Bill is a 38-year-old male from Grenada who lives alone and has suffered from bipolar affective disorder since he was 22 years old. He is unemployed and spends most of his time visiting friends or watching television. He takes lithium carbonate 800 mg to help him control his mood. Although he has no significant past physical medical history, he smokes 30 cigarettes a day and drinks regularly. Lately, he has made frequent visits to his doctor because of a recurrent cough. It transpired that Bill had an upper respiratory tract infection. Before he saw the doctor, the practice nurse took his observations and they were: temperature 37°C; pulse rate 78 beats/min; regular blood pressure (BP) 148/94 mmHg; repeat BP 144/92 mmHg.

We will look at Bill's case later.

The SRM was developed by Leventhal *et al.* (1984) and is built on at least four components:

1. People are active problem solvers and they strive to make sense of their world as they search for suitable, effective ways of controlling and adapting to their world.

2. A multi-level processing system, one emotional and the other intellectual, generates people's perception of health threats.

3. The generation of emotional reactions and the intellectual notions of a disease and its treatment are simultaneous.

4. Contextual factors, including cultural, environmental, social relationships and personality dispositions, influence the way individuals understand health threats and how they manage them. For example, the fact that Bill is of Grenadian origin and lives alone shapes his understanding of health threats.

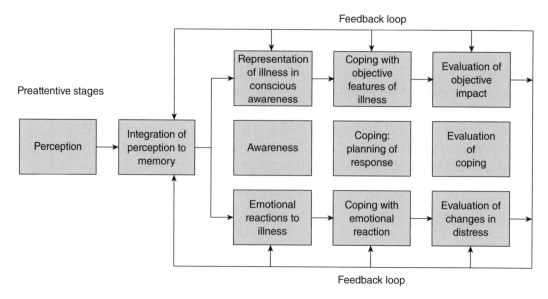

Figure 3.2: Decision-making process according to the Self-Regulation Model. (Adapted from Leventhal et al. 1984)

The use of the SRM is currently widespread, mainly because of its reliability and validity in exploring important patient beliefs across a range of physical illnesses. This allows advances to be made in understanding self-management and recovery of illnesses. Its wide applicability suggests that it may be appropriate for both mental and physical illness.

As we previously mentioned, the SRM was conceptualised by Leventhal and colleagues examining how fear messages in serious situations might lead people to take health-promoting actions, such as wearing seat belts or giving up smoking. Leventhal *et al.* (1984) found that people need different types of information to influence attitudes and actions when they perceive a threat to health and well-being. In this regard, the SRM proposes that, during illness, two parallel processes are in operation: the first is the intellectual or objective interpretation of the threat to health. The second is the emotional or subjective reaction to the threat to health. These parallel processes of intellectual and emotion are interactive.

In the case of Bill, he bases his decision to seek help from his GP from his intellectual processing of information to understand the complex relationship between seeking medical help and the diminishing of persistent coughing. However, socio-culturally related emotional values about illness and seeking help may be more important than intellectual processes. In such situations, people may choose not to seek medical help as they may feel socially obliged not to do so. Before you proceed further with this chapter, you need to take part in this activity.

Activity 3.4   *Reflection*

Read again the case study of Bill. What are the emotional and cultural factors that may influence his decision to seek medical help?

The key beliefs we identify in the SRM refer to a specific illness episode rather than to intellectual beliefs about a potential illness occurrence. In applying the SRM to people with mental health problems with physical illness, we can identify four specific components that are central to guiding an individual's reaction to the threat to health. These are:

1. their perception of the nature of the illness (including a label and signs/symptoms);
2. their perception of the consequences of the illness (physical, social and behavioural);
3. the likely causes of the illness;
4. the likely timeline or sense of how long the illness will last.

A fifth belief we can identify is about the person's perception of potential for control or cure of the illness (Lau *et al.* 1989).

There has been considerable support for the model since its inception. For example, how individuals summarise and label these experiences may have an important impact on their responses and this links to perceived quality of life. Mechanic *et al.* (1994) found that people who attributed their mental illness to a physical, medical or biological problem, as opposed to psychological problems, scored higher on a perceived quality-of-life measure, and reported less personal stigma and greater self-esteem. In addition, the dimension of the likely consequences of having a health problem on daily life correlates with variations in coping levels, depression and health-seeking behaviour.

Overall, evidence suggests that the SRM is a potentially useful way for understanding health-seeking behaviour.

Finally, it is important for you to recognise that we use models to increase our understanding of people's responses to health as tools to help us in potentially important areas of intervention. These conceptualisations have limitations and cannot replace a specific individual's own view of illness which provides a far more complex and useful guide to an understanding of their illness and what it means for him or her. In order to apply these theories in practice, you need to build a working relationship or therapeutic alliance with your patient, and it is this we look at next.

The therapeutic alliance

In the classical medical relationship, the person receiving the help is the patient but the person making the decision is the doctor. We then expect the patient to comply with the doctor's orders as a passive recipient of help. Further, the doctor decides who is sick by providing the patient with a sick certificate; in turn, we expect the sick person to adopt a sick role. Unfortunately, this paternalistic (or authoritarian) approach is fraught with problems. In addition, the growth of consumerism means that patients are increasingly taking an active part in their treatment. More importantly, there is research evidence suggesting that people who play an active role in their treatment are more likely to recover much quicker compared to those who take a passive role. As a mental health nurse, you will need to establish a therapeutic relationship or alliance with your patient as this is a basic tenet of your practice

(Mutsatsa 2011). The therapeutic alliance is an essential tool that facilitates effective care. So what is a therapeutic alliance?

We normally describe the therapeutic alliance as a patient's capacity to collaborate productively with the therapist because the patient sees the therapist as a helping professional with good intentions. In other words, we generally view the therapeutic alliance as involving an agreement between therapist and patient on the goals of treatment, the tasks needed to accomplish those goals and a sense of a personal bond between therapist and patient.

The debate surrounding the therapeutic alliance has been ongoing for nearly a century in the psychotherapy literature. Historically, it was the first concept to be developed in order to capture the special role performed by the patient–psychotherapist relationship. In 1912, Freud outlined the first references to the therapeutic alliance by highlighting its importance as a vehicle for success in psychoanalysis. Some authors even state that the quality of the therapeutic alliance is more important than the type of psychotherapy in predicting positive therapeutic outcomes (Safran 1996). For example, one study compared four groups of 225 individuals with depression having interpersonal psychotherapy, cognitive behavioural therapy (CBT), medication with clinical management, or placebo with clinical management. The study found that the quality of the therapeutic alliance accounted for most of the variance in treatment outcome, regardless of the kind of therapy (Krupnick *et al.* 1996). As a result, the suggestion is that the therapeutic alliance is a prerequisite for all therapies.

In terms of physical health promotion, there is evidence to suggest that a relatively strong therapeutic alliance during the opening phase of an intervention may be the best predictor of good outcome. However, you need to work towards developing this alliance.

Developing a therapeutic alliance

As a nurse, you should help to foster a positive alliance with patients by identifying with their health goals and with the healthy aspects of their self that are striving to reach those goals. Patients will then experience the nurse as a collaborator who is working with them rather than against them. In other words, developing a good alliance with patients will require you not only to be positive and empathetic, but also to work within a collaborative framework, a partnership in which patients see themselves as respected participants (Mutsatsa 2011).

It is important to collaborate with the patient to identify mutually agreed health promotion goals and view the patient as a key stakeholder in the treatment-planning process. You should focus on sharing the decision making between the patient and yourself in order to determine the most appropriate course of action and listen to patients with empathy in order to build a strong relationship with them. This involves identifying their concerns regarding health and addressing any barriers to good health that you jointly identify. By building a strong alliance, you support patients' empowerment, and patients, in turn, will be more likely to adhere to established health promotion. Patients and nurses do not always agree on risk factors for poor health. By discussing patients' perceptions regarding their health, you have the opportunity to address patient concerns without assuming they already know the barriers that may be contributing to their health problems.

> ### Scenario
>
> *Cathy suffers from schizophrenia and has recently been diagnosed with type 2 diabetes but attributes the symptoms of diabetes to evil spirits.*

In people with psychosis like Cathy in the scenario, establishing rapport can be challenging because of the nature of their illness. However, a therapeutic alliance with a patient increases the likelihood that the patient will adhere to specific health-promoting strategies and achieve a better outcome. In his discussion of the therapeutic alliance, Gabbard (2005) noted that mental health professionals ought to be innovative and find some common ground with patients in areas such as music, film, holiday places and sports. If you can identify common interests it will provide an opportunity for the therapeutic relationship to grow. If the patient expresses delusions, it may not be wise to challenge these, but you should view them as metaphors that can shed insight into the patient's inner conflicts. A detailed review on how to communicate with someone with delusions is beyond the scope of this chapter. Please consult an appropriate text on psychosis.

One way of fostering an alliance is to focus on a patient's strengths and accept bizarre behaviour, feelings and thoughts that others do not understand, without judgement. As the alliance develops, you may work with the patient to identify specific issues that cause the patient to relapse and help prevent relapse.

We have seen that engaging patients with schizophrenia in a therapeutic alliance can be difficult. The process can take up to 6 months, and as a nurse, you should not become pessimistic if the patient is not engaging in a collaborative therapeutic relationship after several months. Based on the results discussed by Frank and Gunderson (1990), if an alliance has not formed after 6 months, you may need to re-evaluate the intervention you have agreed with your patient.

Intervention strategies for physical health promotion

It is now widely accepted that poor physical health plays a negative role in the treatment and recovery of people with mental health problems. Interventions such as psychotherapy have proved to be successful as part of health-promoting strategies.

Several intervention strategies can be used, such as alliance building, education, psychotherapy and/or CBT. In this section we will take a brief look at these strategies.

Psychotherapy

Psychological counselling may produce an emotional improvement that can increase the desire and ability of some patients to improve self-care. This is particularly so for those who are depressed, and there is some evidence to support the use of psychotherapy to improve physical health in those with mental health problems. We assume that, by coming to understand their treatment rights and responsibilities, patients can break the cycle of an unfavourable health lifestyle. Psychotherapy is likely to improve feelings of self-worth and independence and this may improve self-efficacy (see earlier sections). For example, a randomised controlled study of 265 patients found that a third of patients could maintain or improve weight loss by inpatient psychotherapy. Other beneficial changes were lasting changes in body image and reduction in distress (Wiltink *et al.* 2007).

Another intervention strategy we can use to improve physical health is health education.

Health education

The WHO has defined health education as *comprising consciously constructed opportunities for learning involving some form of communication designed to improve health literacy, including improving knowledge, and developing life skills which are conducive to individual and community health* (World Health Organization 1998). In other words, health education is about teaching patients all about health (physical and mental). When we teach people with mental health problems about mental illness, we call this psychoeducation. Health education is also a way of accessing and learning strategies to deal with physical health challenges and their effects. It remains a consistently popular tool for intervention for families and carers, as it enables them to make sense of what is happening. For example, a meta-analysis of 52 studies that used Self-Management Education interventions to help people with type 2 diabetes achieve and maintain healthy blood glucose levels recorded a positive role for educational strategies (Klein *et al.* 2013).

Many educational strategies involve individual or group counselling sessions and/or use of written and audiovisual materials on health promotion strategies. For maximum benefit, we should use health education in conjunction with therapies such as CBT.

Cognitive behavioural therapy

CBT is a talking therapy that emphasises the importance of finding new ways of thinking and behaving to deal with current problems. For example, in promoting exercise, an intervention with a CBT base helps patients to question their automatic thoughts about physical exercise. We help patients to mentally connect physical exercise to their improvement in physical health and well-being. In essence, CBT aims to help patients to reduce negative thoughts by changing the way they think about things. The trained therapist generally follows a programme manual and has several individual sessions with patients.

There are instances where a nurse can apply CBT-based principles to help the patient overcome difficulties. For instance, the patient may present with distressing psychiatric symptoms that may be an obstacle to an ongoing health promotion programme to a nurse. In this case, the first and most desirable option is to assist the patient to deal with these, applying CBT informed principles. More likely, you will need to refer the patient to a psychologist or CBT therapist. There is sufficient evidence supporting the use of CBT in improving physical health through exercise promotion (Pimenta *et al.* 2012), smoking cessation (Clarke *et al.* 2013) and a whole host of other conditions (Hofmann *et al.* 2012). Other behavioural approaches to improve physical health include conditioning, rewards, cues, reminders and skills training. These interventions seek to promote, modify and reinforce behaviours related to physical health. Therapists often combine CBT with motivational interviewing (MI) principles for maximum effect.

Motivational interviewing

MI is a directive, client-centred counselling style for stimulating behaviour change in people by helping them to explore and resolve **ambivalence**. In practice, this means that the content of the session centres on the individual's viewpoint (i.e., is person-centred). In addition, the therapist uses the spirit of MI to guide the discussion in the direction of behaviour change (directive) through the resolution of ambivalence. In this regard, the focus on the resolution of ambivalence is central and the therapist is deliberately directive in following this objective. MI has many applications in the health field, including treating addictions. Before we go further, we need to discuss the concept of motivation within the context of MI.

Case study

Ron is a 55-year-old man who suffers from schizophrenia and was diagnosed with coronary heart disease 2 years ago. He lives alone and smokes about 20 cigarettes a day. Ron has tried to give up smoking on several occasions – without success. Lately, Ron has noticed that he has difficulty walking short distances without getting breathless. He also has suffered from recurring chest infections. Although he takes his prescribed medication regularly, he has no energy and does not prepare fresh, healthy foods.

Motivation

It is easy to confuse lack of motivation with lack of activity, but the two are different. For example, a person may have an inner desire to stop smoking (such as Ron in the case study), but fail to achieve this for a variety of reasons. Equally, a person may stop smoking due to external factors without having the desire to stop and therefore when these external factors disappear, the person may start smoking again. To put this differently, you can change people's behaviour by applying external punitive actions if they smoke. The person is likely to stop smoking but is also likely to smoke again once you stop the punitive action.

A more lasting approach is to motivate individuals so that they make a decision for themselves that they want to stop smoking. This desire or intrinsic motivation to stop smoking will still be present in spite of the availability of cigarettes or pressure from other people to smoke. Your role as a nurse is to apply these principles to support and encourage patients through the process of behaviour change, and this requires specific skills.

Collaboration

A collaborative approach is at the heart of MI and is one that emphasises working together with your patient as equal partners in a relationship that is supportive and conducive of change. The relationship should not be, or be perceived to be, coercive. During the collaborative process, an awareness of your own motives, values and views is vital in ensuring that you do not impose these on others.

Another useful and necessary skill of MI is evocation.

Evocation

Evocation is about your own skills as a nurse to listen to, understand and remind patients of their own reasons for change. Although you may have your own view why patients should change their behaviour, the emphasis here is exploring your patient's own knowledge, efforts and motivation to change. This involves eliciting information from the individual rather than imparting knowledge, insight or reality.

Useful approaches might include **Socratic questioning**, exploring ambivalence without judgement by presenting both sides of the decisional balance – and avoiding giving an unsolicited opinion. You should notice, reflect and ask questions to elaborate on **change talk**. It is important to ask the patient questions from a perspective of curiosity rather than from a position of assumption, as this might run the risk of giving the impression that you are advancing a particular viewpoint or interrogating the patient.

In addition to evocation, you should emphasise autonomy in and support the patient.

Autonomy and support

A key element of MI is that the responsibility for change lies with your patient. It is important to respect patients' free will and autonomy at all times. Your main aim is to understand patients' arguments for change and then support them.

In addition to autonomy and support, the provision of direction plays an important role in MI.

Direction

You should honour all of the above principles and approaches while still moving in the direction of change to deliver a directed intervention without confrontation, education or authority. This should occur through careful listening, summarising, affirming and reflecting on just the right information in the person's own words, emphasising their own intent, reason or need for change, and their hope and optimism in achieving this.

Part of providing direction should initially involve assessing readiness to change.

Assessing readiness to change

Several factors influence the behaviour of an individual during the change process. These are desire, ability, reason, need for change and commitment to change. We generally apply the acronym DARNC:

- desire;
- ability;
- reason;
- need for change;
- commitment to change.

You will need to assess these aspects of motivation when you talk with patients. You can assess how your patients are feeling and thinking about changing their current behaviour. For some people, this may involve a lengthy discussion. For others, who are ready to act, for example, you may only hold a brief assessment before planning action. We will look at these factors in turn.

Desire for change

This pertains to how much the patient wants to change. It is what the patient wants to do regardless of logic, need or reason. For example, if Ron has no desire to change, he may want to continue smoking whether cigarettes are available to him or not. This is because Ron may not have that deep-down desire to change his current behaviour. This is important, because desire guides change.

In addition to having the desire for change, the patient has to have the ability to change behaviour.

Ability to change

A patient like Ron may be already thinking about change, but it is still important to assess the patient's ability to change and *beliefs* about this ability. This is because, though most people are able to change their behaviour, they may face real or imaginary obstacles that may undermine their efforts to change. In people with mental health problems, real obstacles may include cognitive deficits such as poor memory which may prevent them from effecting behaviour change. In some cases, the use of substances such as cannabis, alcohol and others can have a negative impact on the memory and thinking, creating an obstacle for change. In other instances, psychotropic medication can induce side effects such as drowsiness, restlessness, constipation and many more, which may interfere with ability to effect change.

Another area of real obstacles is the patient's social circumstances. It is important to assess the patient's social circumstances, as some patients may experience peer or family pressure to continue with current behaviour.

Apart from real obstacles, patients may face belief obstacles in their quest for change.

Belief obstacles are those beliefs that undermine a plan for change. For example, Ron might believe that he is unable to stop smoking because he does not have the willpower. *Belief* obstacles become firmer when previous experiences seem to support that viewpoint. In Ron's case, the belief obstacle may be firmer due to his previous attempts to stop smoking that ended in failure. To help your patients to overcome this, you need to acknowledge their previous attempts to change behaviour and reframe this as partially successful. This helps to minimise failure beliefs that patients might have and strengthens beliefs about their ability. It is also important to assess why the patient wants to change behaviour to gain a more rounded view.

Reason for change

Consider a situation where you're treating a patient like Ron, who acknowledges that he smokes excessively and that this damages his health. Ron may feel there is a need to give up smoking. However, he also feels that he does not have a good reason for giving up smoking because he believes there are many other things that contribute to poor health and giving up smoking will not make any difference. Besides, Ron feels that smoking helps him relax and socialise. Further, the reason for change interacts with the need for change, which we will turn to next.

Need for change

In some cases, a patient may not express a desire to stop smoking but can clearly identify problems with continued smoking behaviour. For example, Ron may link smoking to his recurrent chest infection. This does not mean that Ron is ready to act or will change. Therefore, Ron has a *desire* to continue smoking but a *need* to change behaviour because of smoking-related respiratory illness. The respiratory illness is potentially a *need* to change and the patient acknowledges the advantages and disadvantages of behaviour change. The patient may be *ambivalent* to change or *contemplate change* because of a *desire* to continue smoking. The patient may react by denying the need to change behaviour and become *pre-contemplative* (see the transtheoretical model of change, above). Therefore, you need to distinguish between need and desire to change.

Commitment to change

This is where your patient wants to put in the necessary effort to change and sustain these changes. In general, factors that influence commitment are the desire, ability, reason and need for change (DARN).

Therapeutic skills required for MI

When you are using MI, you should use four major skills of intervention, which we remember using the acronym OARS:

1. Ask *open*-ended questions.
2. *Affirm* patients' self-efficacy.
3. *Reflect* on patients' thoughts via active listening.
4. *Summarise* patients' narratives to help resolve ambivalence and promote change.

Let us look at these now in turn.

Open-ended questions

Right from the beginning, you should let the patient do most of the talking during therapy, as this allows you to shape the patient's speech such as eliciting change talk. You should ask a mixture of closed and open questions. Closed questions are those that a person can answer with a short simple phrase or word, or yes or no. For example, 'How old are you?' and 'Where are you going?' are closed questions. Closed questions tend to give you facts, are easy and quick to answer and you can keep control of the conversation.

In contrast, open questions encourage patients to explain or expand their answer. Open-ended question tend to start with What? Why? or How? For example, 'What did you do on Christmas day?' 'How did you manage to do all that work in an hour?' We frame open-ended questions in such a way as to encourage further discussion. They have the following characteristics: they ask the patient to think and reflect, will give you the opinions and feelings of the patient, and will hand control of the conversation over to the patient. In this respect, they encourage the patient to open up. You should avoid asking more than three questions in a row: you can intersperse question with reflections, affirmations and summaries (see following sections).

Affirmations

At its most basic definition, an affirmation refers to positive mental attitude and self-efficacy. These can include the positive statements a patient makes about changing behaviour. You need to recognise these as encouraging without being excessive in your acknowledgement. Sometimes it can be worth checking back on how the comments feel to the individual.

Reflective listening

This is a communication approach that involves two key stages. The first stage is to try to understand the patient's point of view. The second important stage is that you should offer the point of view back to the patient to confirm that you understood it correctly. In other words, you attempt to 'reconstruct' what the patient is thinking and feeling and then communicate this understanding back to the patient. To be effective in reflective listening, you should be able to step back from the words and think about alternative meanings of the spoken words. In reflective listening, you are checking out whether the meaning that you guessed is correct before moving forward.

Another skill you need in MI is summarising and we will turn to this next.

Summarising

The main purpose of summarising is to link information together, recap and reinforce important change talk from the patient. In summaries, we can collect information together and then conclude with an open encouragement to the patient. Summaries can link different information, such as the two sides of ambivalence, which you can better link by 'and' or 'at the same time', which emphasise the ambivalence, rather than 'but' or 'yet', which can be more confusing. For example, you may say, 'So, on one hand, you have concerns about how much you smoke and on the other hand you have worries about how out of breath you get when you walk very far *and* at the same time smoking is one of your few pleasures in life.'

Express empathy

Empathy is the experience of understanding another person's condition from the patient's point of view. When you express empathy, you place yourself in the other person's shoes and imagine, to the best of your ability, what s/he is feeling. There is evidence suggesting that empathy increases helping behaviours (prosocial). In this respect, accurate empathy or 'acceptance' is the process of seeking to understand and accept your patient's feelings and point of view through skilful reflective listening. You do not need to agree with the patient; it is possible for you to have a different view from the patient, and you can still express that view if the patient asks you. You should however be able to respect the fact that the patient asked you while at the same time having a respect for the patient's own different stance. This approach is likely to help you to build collaboration, while promoting a sense of autonomy in the patient.

Develop discrepancy

The aim of developing discrepancy is to draw your patient's attention to the difference between where the patient is now and where s/he ideally wants to be in terms of change. For example, if your patient's life goal is to improve his or her physical health, then there is a potential disparity between his or her smoking behaviour and this health goal. You may develop discrepancy by prompting your patient to consider the cost of his or her current behaviour (e.g. breathlessness when going upstairs) and the benefit of change (e.g. more energy during exercise) and relate these to the chance of achieving the lifetime goal of being healthy. The greater the importance the patient attaches to a life goal (e.g. to be physically healthy) and the greater the discrepancy between this goal and current behaviour (e.g. smoking), the more likely your patient will move towards change. You just need to be careful that the goals are the patient's, not yours. Every patient has different life experiences and skills. Some patients may need to make more changes in comparison to others to reach the same goal (e.g. smoking cessation).

Avoid argument

It is not acceptable to try to force or argue for a behaviour change in patients because in doing so, they are more likely to argue for things to remain as they are. You may offer new information and a new perspective to patients but you should do this with patients' agreement that they can take it or leave it.

In addition to avoiding argument, rolling with resistance is critical.

Roll with resistance

If you meet with resistance, you should not see this as a negative development on the part of the patient; rather it is a sign that your conversation with the patient is perhaps proceeding far too quickly. Instead of fighting this resistance, which may develop into an argument, one way of overcoming it is to respond differently by reframing this resistance and actively involve the patient in problem solving while respecting the patient's autonomy. Patients can be seen to have the answers to their problems and the nurse should focus on asking questions rather than answering them.

An approach that focuses on answering a patient's questions may encourage the patient to find fault with these answers. For example, if you face a question such as, 'What do you think I should do about my smoking then?', an inappropriate response might be: 'Well, I think if you stop smoking, it always helps with your health.' The patient might find fault in this and may respond, 'Yes, but smoking is the only enjoyable thing I do in my day.' Instead, you should elicit reasons why your patient wants to continue smoking. Alternatively, you can give a response that emphasises the patient's own ability to answer the question. For example, you could say, 'I think that you know more about your situation than I do and you're good at coming up with ideas as to what to do', or 'I am just wondering, what ideas do you have?' This type of response promotes self-efficacy and encourages change talk in the patient.

Support self-efficacy

We have described self-efficacy as the belief individuals have in their ability to change or overcome difficulties. Your own belief in patients' ability to change behaviour should enhance their self-efficacy. You should demonstrate this by emphasising any success the patient might have had in overcoming obstacles. Without this belief, the patient is unlikely to change behaviour, as any change needs to come from the individual and not from external others. Patients are likely to change behaviour if they are getting support from carers.

Carer involvement

As discussed previously, families can have an impact on patients' desire to take part in health promotion strategies. Family members with negative attitudes to health promotion and other misconceptions about the nature of their loved ones' physical and mental health can be a barrier to a healthy lifestyle (Julius *et al.* 2009). Research evidence demonstrates health improvement in those patients whose family members are actively engaged in their care and who receive some level of intervention by mental health professionals. With the patient's permission, you should involve family members in treatment planning and addressing potential concerns about recommended treatment. You should also involve relatives in providing educational information to the patient about the physical illness, its treatment and prevention. It is also important to identify and discuss families' ability and willingness to support the patient and encourage healthy living and to recommend treatments.

It is also important to provide emotional support to families to enable them to cope with the physical and mental illness of their loved one. For example, you might encourage family members to participate in local support groups, such as those sponsored by voluntary organisations (Julius *et al.* 2009).

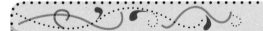

Chapter summary

According to WHO, health is a state of complete physical, mental and social well-being and not merely the absence of disease or infirmity. Health plays a central role in people's lives and it is important for you to acknowledge its multidimensional nature. With this in mind, we need to develop strategies for promoting health in people with mental health problems. Health promotion is the process of enabling people to increase control over, and to improve, their health in order to reach a

continued . . .

state of complete physical, mental and social well-being. To be able to do this, we need to utilise strategies that have their origins in health-promoting theories. Some of these theories are the Health Belief Model, the SRM, transtheoretical, and Self-Efficacy Models. Some therapies, such as psychotherapy and CBT, enhance health and health promotion. To be effective, health promotion intervention strategies should be underpinned by a good therapeutic alliance and communication skills that incorporate principles of MI.

Activities: brief outline answers

Activity 3.1

Being healthy is not merely the absence of a disease. Moreover, health is not an all-or-nothing issue. Rather, it exists on a continuum where one end is the complete absence of physical and mental disease and the other end is the presence of disease.

Activity 3.2

The measures you take should be guided by Kofi's wishes. He should have a sense of ownership of the decision-making process. You could suggest several ways of losing weight without spending too much money.

Activity 3.3

No. Her view of illness is perfectly valid when one considers her cultural background. In Ayurveda (Indian traditional medicine) it is the norm to believe that illness is a result of a lack of balance between *vāta, pitta* and *kapha.*

Activity 3.4

Persistent coughing is likely to be irritating or even painful. From a socio-cultural perspective, his friends or family might pressurise him to see a doctor or those close to him might generally seek medical help when they are coughing a lot; therefore he is obliged to see one as well when he has the same condition.

Further reading

Green J, Tones K (2010) *Health Promotion, Planning and Strategies.* London: SAGE.

This is a comprehensive book on health promotion and theories relating to health promotion.

Miller WR, Rollnick S (2012) *Motivational Interviewing,* 3rd edn. *Helping People Change (Applications of Motivational Interviewing).* New York: Guilford Press.

This is a very good book on motivational interviewing.

Useful websites

http://www.who.int/topics/health_promotion/en

This World Health Organization website is useful as it provides up-to-date policies on health promotion matters.

http://www.motivationalinterview.org/index.html

This MI site has material that facilitates the dissemination, adoption and implementation of MI among clinicians, supervisors, programme managers and trainers, and improves treatment outcomes for clients with substance use disorders.

www.healthpromotion.org.uk

This site was designed mainly to support those working in the areas of health promotion and public health. The information is also of interest and use to professionals from a range of other sectors, as well as students and interested members of the public.

Chapter 4
The care and management of cardiovascular disorders

Chapter aims

By the end of the chapter, you should be able to:

- understand and describe the cardiovascular group of diseases;
- discuss the risk factors associated with various cardiovascular conditions;
- discuss primary, secondary and tertiary interventions for cardiovascular disorders.

Introduction

Cardiovascular disease (CVD) is an umbrella term that includes diseases of the heart, stroke (cerebrovascular disease), high blood pressure (hypertension), peripheral arterial disease, rheumatic, heart and congestive cardiac disease. According to the World Health Organization (WHO), CVD is the number one cause of death globally. In other words, more people die annually from CVD than from any other cause (WHO 2011a). Current estimates are that 17.3 million people died from CVD in 2008 alone and this figure represents 30% of all global deaths. In the same report, the WHO asserts that CVD disproportionately affects people from low- to middle-income countries. More worryingly, research evidence suggests that the number of people likely to die from CVD will increase, to reach 23.3 million by 2030 (Mathers and Loncar 2006). In 2007, CVD caused over 190,000 deaths in the UK, accounting for 40% of all deaths. More than 4 million people have suffered from CVD and it costs the UK approximately £30 billion annually (Luengo-Fernandez *et al.* 2006). Clearly CVD poses a serious public health problem and the risk of developing CVD in people with mental health problems is significantly higher than in the general population, as we discussed in Chapter 1.

Cardiovascular disease and mental health

Case study

Gary is a 47-year-old male born in London of Jamaican parentage. Gary has suffered from depression since he lost his job at the age of 33. He has been taking imipramine 75 mg at night and he was diagnosed with hypertension 4 years ago. He smokes 20 cigarettes a day and saw his doctor recently; the GP conducted tests which were all unremarkable except for his body mass index (BMI), which was 30 kg/m^2; his weight circumference ratio was 102 cm (40 inches), resting blood pressure 144/80 mmHg and total cholesterol 6 mmol/L.

Evidence suggests that people with mental health problems such as schizophrenia, depression and bipolar disorder are three times more likely to die from CVD in comparison to the general population. In fact, the commonest cause of death in this group is CVD (Brown *et al.* 2009). There is increasing evidence suggesting that mental illnesses such as schizophrenia, depression and anxiety are independent risk factors for the development of CVD (Khayyam-Nekouei *et al.* 2013). People with schizophrenia have a higher mean 10-year CVD risk of 4.6%, in comparison with the general population of 3.1%. In addition, evidence in support of an association between depression and coronary heart disease (CHD) (Sachdev 1995) has been accumulating over the last two decades. The prevalence of depression in patients with heart failure is 20% higher than in healthy individuals (Kuper *et al.* 2002).

There are many reasons why people with mental health problems are vulnerable to CVD. We discussed some of these factors in Chapter 1 but, briefly, people with mental health problems are more likely to be overweight, to smoke, and to have diabetes, hypertension and dyslipidaemia. They are more likely to have a family history of diabetes and there is an association between mental illness and the chronic elevations of stress hormones. More importantly, the treatment of mental health disorders with psychotropic medication poses a huge risk to patients both in terms of direct effect on the cardiovascular system and indirectly through inducing weight gain. These factors directly or indirectly alter the anatomy and physiology of the cardiovascular system and we will discuss these risk factors in more detail in later sections. We will now turn to the abnormal anatomy and physiology of the cardiovascular system.

The anatomy and physiology of the cardiovascular system and its pathology

The main components of the human cardiovascular system are the heart, blood and the blood vessels, as shown in Figure 4.1. The main function of this system is for the blood to transport oxygen, hormones, proteins and nutrients such as glucose to different parts of body tissues. This enables the body to function normally.

An additional function of the cardiovascular system is to transport metabolic waste such as carbon dioxide to the lungs and urea and other waste to the kidneys and skin for expulsion from the body. To be able to function properly, an average adult's cardiovascular system should contain about 6 litres of blood, accounting for roughly 7% of adult body weight. More importantly, to enable efficient blood transportation, the vessels should be more elastic, as vessel dilation allows more blood transport. Unfortunately, in CVD, atherosclerosis compromises the efficient transportation of blood. Atherosclerosis is a disease in which plaque or atheroma builds up

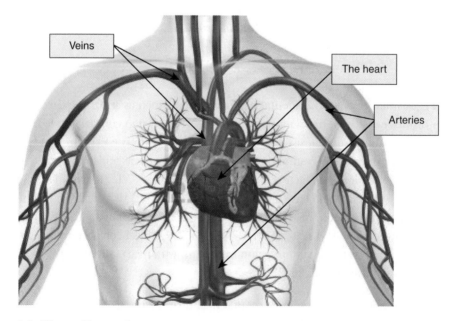

Figure 4.1: The cardiovascular system

inside the walls of the arteries. This plaque is an aggregation of fat, cholesterol, calcium, platelets and other substances found in the blood. There is much debate about the exact cause of atherosclerosis. However, research shows that it is a slow, complex disease that may start in childhood. It develops faster as we age and starts when certain factors damage the inner layers of the arteries. These factors include smoking, high amounts of fats, high blood pressure and high amounts of sugar in the blood. Over time, the plaque hardens and narrows the arteries and this limits the flow of oxygen-rich blood to the organs and other parts of the body (Figure 4.2).

Before you proceed further, please take part in the activity below.

Activity 4.1   *Evidence-based practice and research*

In a group or on your own, research the prevalence of sleep disorders in people with mental health problems. Find out how these contribute to the development of CVD.

There are outline answers to all the activities at the end of the chapter.

Risk factors for the development of cardiovascular disease

You should assess all patients for modifiable risk factors for the development of CVD on first referral; this applies to all patients with mental health problems under your care. Patients suffering from psychosis pose a particular challenge in terms of assessment. Psychosis disrupts communication so patients may not readily provide you with accurate information. One way of overcoming this is to use the Framingham risk score (Zomer *et al.* 2011). This tool identifies many risk factors for the development of CVD, the most common of which we will look at now.

Unhealthy blood cholesterol levels

Cholesterol is a waxy, fat-like substance that the liver produces and is vital for normal body function. The body needs cholesterol to make hormones, vitamin D and other substances that help with digestion. Cholesterol travels through the blood stream in small packages made of fat (lipid) on the inside and proteins on the outside, hence their name, lipoproteins. The body needs to have correct levels of cholesterol travelling in lipoproteins and there are two types.

We call the first type of cholesterol low-density lipoprotein (LDL-C), or 'bad' cholesterol in common parlance. This is because LDL-C drives the development and progression of atherosclerosis in the arteries. Therefore, it is preferable to have lower levels of LDL-C, as this lowers the risk of developing atherosclerosis. High-density lipoprotein cholesterol (HDL-C) or 'good' cholesterol is the second type that we find in our blood. It is good cholesterol because it transports cholesterol from the arteries back to the liver for removal from the body or for reusage. Individuals with high levels of HDL-C seem to have fewer problems with CVD, while those with low HDL-C have

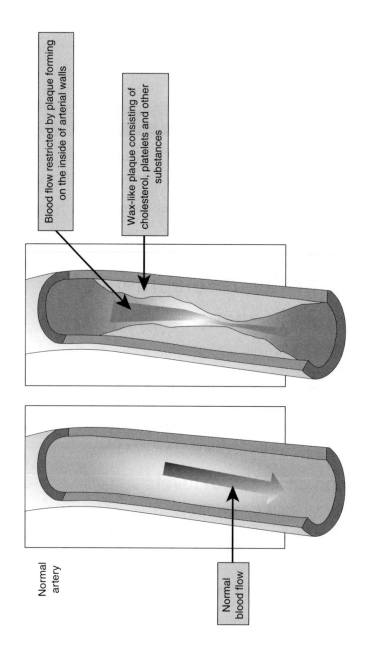

Blood flow restricted by plaque forming on the inside of arterial walls

Wax-like plaque consisting of cholesterol, platelets and other substances

Normal artery

Normal blood flow

Figure 4.2: Cutaway of an artery with plaque and one without

increased rates of heart disease (Toth 2005). More importantly, increasing HDL-C through good dietary intake improves cardiovascular health (Haffner 2004). Poor dietary intake that is deficient in HDL-C and rich in LDL-C is not uncommon in people with mental health problems (Stanley and Laugharne 2014).

In summary, the higher the level of LDL-C in your blood, the greater the chance of getting CVD; conversely, the higher the level of HDL-C in your blood, the lower your chances of getting CVD. In practice, you should discuss with your patients to address those factors that promote high LDL-C and low HDL-C. However, for many patients with mental health problems, lifestyle modification may not be enough to achieve adequate elevations in HDL-C as heredity plays an important role in regulating the level of HDL-C. Mutations in one or more genes can give some people a very high level of HDL-C and predispose others to very low levels of HDL-C. Many patients will require the combination of medication with lifestyle modification and we will discuss this in later sections.

The second risk factor for the development of atherosclerosis is high blood pressure and we will turn to this next. Before we proceed, please take part in the activity below.

Activity 4.2   *Evidence-based practice and research*

HDL-Cs are very important for our health. Alone or in a group, find out about ways of raising HDL-C in the body.

High blood pressure

We define high blood pressure or hypertension as a systolic blood pressure at or above 140 mmHg and/or a diastolic blood pressure at or above 90 mmHg (see Chapter 2).

In comparison with normal blood pressure at the same age, hypertension significantly increases the risk of CVD threefold. Hypertension accelerates the formation of atherosclerosis (atherogenesis) and therefore promotes premature coronary disease. It puts the body's blood vessels under stress, causing them to clog or weaken. It also makes the blood vessels more likely to block from blood clots or parts of the plaque to break off from the lining of the blood vessel wall. If there is damage to the arteries, this can create weak places that can rupture easily or create thin spots that cause the artery wall to balloon out (aneurysm). We normally associate hypertension in people under 50 years old with elevated risk of CVD. As we get older, systolic blood pressure becomes a more important predictor of the risk of CVD. People who suffer from serious mental illness in particular are prone to hypertension.

It follows that people with hypertension tend to have high levels of LDL-C and low levels of HDL-C. In addition, they suffer impairment in glucose tolerance (see Chapter 5) and ECG abnormalities. Those at risk for hypertensive stroke have an enlarged left ventricle or left ventricular hypertrophy, atrial fibrillation, cardiac failure, coronary disease, diabetes or a cigarette habit.

We now need to look at smoking as a specific risk factor for CVD.

Smoking

Smoking is a major risk factor for the development of heart disease, in tandem with other risk factors such as unhealthy blood cholesterol levels, high blood pressure and obesity. Tobacco contains at least 4000 chemicals, some of which harm the blood and other cells in the body. These chemicals can also damage the function of the heart, the structure and function of the blood vessels (see Chapter 7). The injury that smoking inflicts on the cardiovascular system increases the risk of atherosclerosis. Furthermore, smoking is a major risk factor for the development of peripheral arterial disease. This is a condition in which plaque builds up in the arteries that carry blood to the head, organs and limbs. People who have peripheral arterial disease are at high risk of developing heart disease, heart attack or stroke.

Any amount of smoking, even light or occasional smoking, damages the heart and blood vessels. For some people, such as women who use birth control pills and people who have diabetes, smoking poses an even greater risk to the heart and blood vessels. In addition, passive smoking or second-hand smoke can harm the heart and blood vessels. We define second-hand smoke as the involuntary inhaling of smoke from other people's cigarettes, cigars or pipes. Passive smoking contains many of the same harmful chemicals that people inhale when they smoke and damages the heart and blood vessels of people who do not smoke in the same way as active smoking does. Passive smoke also raises children and teenagers' risk of future CVD because it lowers the levels of HDL-C (Toth 2005), raises blood pressure and damages heart tissues. This risk is greater in premature babies with respiratory distress syndrome and asthma. Many patients with mental health problems smoke tobacco and smoking cessation for patients is an important intervention target (see Chapter 5).

Another important risk factor for the development of CVD is insulin resistance.

Insulin resistance

Insulin is a hormone that helps transport blood glucose sugar into cells where it is a source of energy. Insulin resistance is a condition in which the body produces insulin but does not use it effectively. The body's muscle, fat and liver cells do not respond properly to insulin and thus cannot easily absorb glucose from the blood stream. Apart from its direct effect on diabetes, insulin resistance is an independent risk factor for CVD by up to a 2.5-fold increase. Multiple prospective studies have documented an association between insulin resistance and an acceleration in CVD in patients with type 2 diabetes, as well as in non-diabetic individuals (DeFronzo 2010).

Diabetes

Over time, insulin resistance can lead to pre-diabetes and type 2 diabetes because the beta cells (in the pancreas) that make insulin fail to keep up with the body's increasing need for insulin. Without enough insulin, excess glucose builds up in the blood stream, leading to pre-diabetes, diabetes and other serious health disorders.

Healthy and normal blood vessels have an inner lining or endothelium that keeps blood flowing smoothly by producing the gas nitric oxide. Nitric oxide relaxes the smooth muscles in the inner walls of blood vessels and prevents blood cells from sticking to them. It is the disruption of this process that we believe is central to the increase in plaque formation in people with diabetes. High blood sugar, elevated saturated fatty acids and **triglycerides** lead to a stickier inner lining and this encourages the attachment of blood cells. The attachment of blood cells produces local tissue reaction. The local tissue reaction further traps floating particles and different cells, piling up and hardening the vessel walls.

Insulin stimulates the production of nitric oxide by the endothelium cells but this stimulatory effect is lost in people with diabetes and insulin resistance, and these two conditions are common in people with serious mental illness (see Chapter 5). The stimulatory loss results in an increasing tendency towards plaque formation inside the blood vessels. High blood sugar levels and insulin resistance not only reduce the production of nitric oxide, they also increase the production of substances that constrict the blood vessel and therefore further encourage plaque formation. Furthermore, high blood glucose affects platelets and clotting factors by increasing **coagulability** and **fibrinolytic** impairment (Lemkes *et al.* 2010). In people with high blood glucose, the blood cells are much stickier and the factors that inhibit clots (fibrinolytic factors) do not work well in diabetes. As we suggest in Chapter 5, diabetes is common in people with serious mental illness and there is also a relationship between diabetes and obesity, both of which are common in people with serious mental illness.

Overweight or obesity

The terms overweight and obesity refer to body weight that is greater than what we consider healthy for a certain height. There is a strong association between obesity and atherosclerosis (Mauricio *et al.* 2013) and there is coverage of this topic in detail in Chapter 5. There are other miscellaneous factors in addition to the factors mentioned.

Other factors

Other factors which contribute to the build-up of atherosclerosis in the body include lack of physical exercise, unhealthy diet, older age and genetic factors. A lack of physical activity can worsen other risk factors for atherosclerosis, such as unhealthy blood cholesterol levels, high blood pressure, high C-reactive protein (CRP) levels, diabetes, overweight and obesity. We will look at these factors in more detail.

An unhealthy diet that consists of foods rich in saturated *trans*-fats can increase the risk for atherosclerosis. Furthermore, foods rich in sodium and sugar can worsen other atherosclerosis risk factors. In addition, genetic factors cause plaque to build up in the arteries as people age. By the time one reaches middle age or older, enough plaque has built up to cause signs or symptoms. The risk increases after the age of 45 years for men and 55 years for women.

High levels of CRP in the blood may raise the risk for atherosclerosis and heart attack. High levels of CRP are a sign of inflammation, the body's response to injury or infection. In this regard, damage to the arteries' inner walls triggers inflammation and helps plaque to grow. People who have low CRP levels may develop atherosclerosis at a slower rate than people who have high CRP levels. Studies show a clear link between high CRP levels with schizophrenia

(Miller *et al.* 2013), depression (Howren *et al.* 2009) and anxiety (Copeland *et al.* 2012). Taken together, these findings support the assertion that mental illness in itself is a clear risk factor for the development of CHD.

In addition to these risk factors, evidence suggests that the most commonly reported 'trigger' for a heart attack is an emotionally upsetting event, especially one involving anger. Most mental health problems negatively affect emotion, and this can increase cholesterol levels; therefore it is not surprising that CVD like CHD is common is this population. Interventions that target a reduction in negative emotion will subsequently reduce morbidity and mortality due to CHD.

Coronary heart disease

Case study

Judy is a 49-year-old woman who suffers from schizophrenia and has been taking antipsychotics since she was 22 years old. As a result, she gained significant weight and her BMI increased to 28 kg/m². Four years ago, she was diagnosed with hypertension and takes propranolol 40 mg/day. She has frequently told people that she hates exercise because this wakes up a little animal inside her that squeezes her chest and travels to her arms and neck, causing pain. Recently, she was admitted to hospital after feeling breathless and dizzy. Laboratory tests revealed total serum cholesterol 7 mmol/L, HDL-C 1.4 mmol/L, triglycerides 0.88 mmol/L, LDL-C 2.4 mmol/L and fasting blood glucose of 6.4 mmol/L. Judy was later discharged on a drug regimen of aspirin, propranolol, captopril, simvastatin and isosorbide dinitrate.

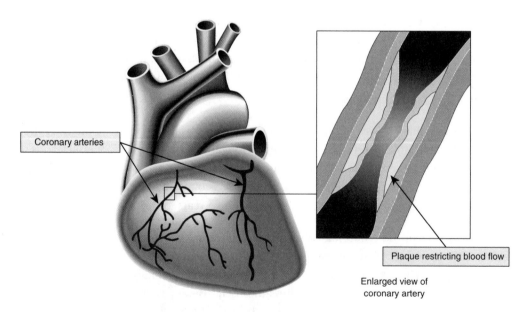

Figure 4.3: The heart and (inset) a coronary artery that is narrowed by plaque

CHD is the leading cause of death worldwide. It occurs when there is insufficient blood supply to the heart muscles. The build-up of plaque on the inner wall of the coronary arteries (Figure 4.3) causes blood supply restriction to the heart's muscles, starving them of oxygen, glucose and other important nutrients. For this reason, the heart cannot work properly and this results in chest pains (O'Donnell *et al.* 2012), as in the case of Judy in the case study. If the plaque completely blocks the coronary artery, it will most likely result in a heart attack.

It is vitally important to remember that many mental illnesses such as schizophrenia affect the person's ability to communicate effectively. At times, what may appear to be delusion is in fact metaphorical expression of an existing problem, as in Judy's case above. Judy believes that exercise wakes a little animal inside her that squeezes her chest. At face value, this explanation may seem a little bizarre but it is intelligible when you consider Judy's health. In other words, it is Judy's metaphorical way of describing her symptoms. Psychiatrists call these types of expression **secondary delusions**. Therefore, you should investigate your patient's complaints thoroughly before you can conclude it is due to altered perception. You will need to recognise the signs and symptoms of CHD and it is to these we now turn.

Signs and symptoms of CHD

The most common symptoms of CHD are angina (chest pain) and myocardial infarction (heart attack). Patients may experience other symptoms, such as palpitations and breathlessness.

Angina

Angina is chest pain or discomfort that occurs if an area of the heart muscle does not get enough oxygen-rich blood. It may feel like pressure or squeezing in the patient's chest. The patient may also feel it in the shoulders, arms, neck, jaw or back. Patients with illness such as schizophrenia may not readily describe these symptoms accurately. For example, Judy describes it as a little animal that travels to the arms and neck, causing pain. Some patients describe angina like indigestion and the pain tends to get worse with activity and go away with rest. Therefore, you need to observe carefully those patients at risk of developing CHD during and after physical activities. Emotional stress also can trigger the angina and again you need to be vigilant in those at risk during periods of heightened emotions. The severity of these symptoms varies and they may get more severe as the coronary arteries continue to narrow due to plaque building up.

Myocardial infarction

As we discussed earlier, a myocardial infarction (heart attack) occurs if there is blood flow blockage to a heart muscle. The blockage can occur if a section of plaque inside the coronary artery ruptures (breaks open). Next, blood platelets will stick to the site of the rupture and aggregate to form a blood clot. If a clot becomes large enough, it can completely block blood flow through a coronary artery. If we do not treat a blood clot, a portion of the heart muscle begins to die due to lack of oxygen and nutrients. Scar tissue replaces healthy heart tissue. Quite often, this heart damage may not be obvious and it may cause severe or long-lasting problems.

In terms of symptoms, the warning signs and symptoms of a myocardial infarction can differ from person to person. Many myocardial infarctions start slowly as mild pain or discomfort. Some people may have myocardial infarctions without any symptoms or very mild symptoms and we call this silent heart attack. In general, most common myocardial infarction symptoms tend to be:

- chest pain or discomfort in the centre or left side of the chest. This pain or discomfort can last for more than a few minutes. Antacids or simple analgesia does not usually relieve the pain and patients say the discomfort can feel like uncomfortable pressure, squeezing, fullness or pain. In some cases, myocardial infarction pain can feel like indigestion or heartburn;

- fatigue, or lack of energy, including sleep problems;

- upper-body discomfort in one or both arms, the back, neck, jaw or upper part of the stomach;

- shortness of breath, which may occur with or before chest discomfort;

- nausea and vomiting, light-headedness or fainting, or breaking out in a cold sweat.

Investigations for myocardial infarction

We normally decide if someone is having a heart attack based on signs and symptoms, personal and family medical history and test results. The test results include electrocardiogram (ECG), blood tests and angiography.

Electrocardiogram

If your patient is complaining of chest pains, it is safe to assume that it is cardiac pain until proven otherwise. In such a case, you need to record the ECG using a 12-lead machine (details of how to record an ECG are given in Chapter 2). If the ECG is normal, this does not mean the cause of the pain is not cardiac but it should ease the panic. In people with pulmonary embolism, sinus rhythm, sinus tachycardia or atrial fibrillation, the ECG may be normal. If you suspect this to be the case, give the patient oxygen, call the doctor and call an ambulance (dial 999). Elevated ST segment may indicate a heart attack, in which case give the patient 300 mg aspirin orally and treat this as an emergency. Monitor and administer oxygen if the oxygen saturation (SpO_2) is low. You should also ensure that the medical emergency box is in close proximity in case it is required. At all times, you should communicate with and reassure the patient, and explain what is happening.

Blood tests

During a heart attack, heart muscle cells die and release proteins into the blood stream. We can measure the amount of these proteins in the blood stream using a **troponin test, CK** or **CK-MB tests** and **serum myoglobin** tests. Higher than normal levels of these proteins suggest a heart attack. As a nurse, you are responsible for coordinating these tests.

Coronary angiography

In coronary angiography, we use a dye and special X-rays to show the inside of the coronary artery to help find blockages during a myocardial infarction. This process requires cardiac catheterisation, where we insert a thin, flexible tube into a blood vessel in the arm, groin or neck. We thread the tube into the coronary arteries and then release a dye into the blood stream. The next step is to take special X-rays while the dye is flowing through the coronary arteries. The dye lets us study the flow of blood through the heart and blood vessels and identifies the site of the blockage.

Primary and secondary prevention of CHD

Prevention is better than cure for any disease. In prevention, we not only focus on measures to prevent the occurrence of a disease such as risk factor reduction, but also to arrest its progress and reduce its consequences once established. In primary prevention you should aim to establish and maintain conditions to minimise hazards to health in general by establishing environmental, economic, social and behavioural conditions conducive for health (see Chapter 9). This approach lies outside the traditional nurse–patient relationship and the medical model. Nevertheless, this social/ecological approach has economic and social benefits for patients outside the health arena, as well as extending cost reduction to diseases other than CHD. It is important to work with the patient in changing the environment that promotes major risk factors for development of CHD.

In some cases, you may need to carry out secondary prevention that generally focuses on the effort to modify risk factors or prevent their development with the aim of delaying or preventing new-onset CHD. Among the strategies we use to lower risk for the development of CHD are re-education, reorientation and motivation of individuals so their lifestyle does not permit risk factors to develop, or to slow down to the extent that their lifetime risk for the development of the disease is low. For example, if we encourage people to lose 15% or more of their body weight, this can drastically reduce the risk of CVD by up to 45% and simultaneously lower CRP levels (Lavie *et al.* 2009). One way of achieving this weight loss is through exercise and improvement in diet, as we discuss in Chapter 9.

Acute care of myocardial infarction

Case study

George is a 57-year-old man who suffers from schizophrenia and lives in the community with his wife. He has been complaining of central 'crushing' chest pain radiating to the neck and shoulders for the past 2 hours. His wife explained that George has been having episodes of 'indigestion' for the last 4 months. The past medical history includes a diagnosis of hypertension 9 years ago and George's father died suddenly of an unknown illness at the age of 55 years. George smokes 20 cigarettes a day and drinks regularly. His care coordinator noticed he was looking unwell, breathless, grey and sweating. His blood pressure was 138/94 mmHg, pulse 96 beats/min regular. The care coordinator contacted the ambulance, which arrived within 5 minutes.

Our immediate concern for a patient we suspect of having a myocardial infarction is for the patient's safety and comfort. This involves the administration of oxygen, analgesia, antiemetics and nitrates. Early treatment for a myocardial infarction can prevent or limit damage to the heart muscle. If you act fast, at the first symptoms of a myocardial infarction, you can save a person's life. You should start certain intervention immediately if you suspect that your patient is having a myocardial infarction, as in the example of George, above. You should ensure that you have a defibrillator and the emergency bag ready in case the patient develops **ventricular fibrillation**. The ambulance service personnel normally have this equipment and it is likely that George was administered oxygen and nitrates by them. If you are on the ward, the action to take should include the following:

- Check the saturated oxygen levels using a pulse oximeter (see Chapter 2) and see if any of the signs below are present:

  1. the patient is unable to talk because of breathlessness;
  2. the patient has fever or lower than usual blood pressure;
  3. the patient experiences pain when breathing with accompanying fast pulse, dizziness and chest pain, as this is an indication that cardiac output has fallen.

  The situation is an emergency and minutes can make a difference, so call for assistance, give oxygen and continue to monitor the SpO_2 rate. Communicate interventions and reassure your patient.

- Give aspirin (300 mg) orally to thin the blood and prevent further blood clotting in the arteries. You should ask the patient to chew and then swallow. The case of George above is a good example of a patient who can potentially benefit from emergency aspirin treatment.

- Give glyceryl trinitrate (GTN) sublingually as it dilates the blood vessels and therefore improves blood flow to the coronary arteries. The pain may settle quickly after GTN has been given, though it may recur. Whilst waiting for assistance, you can do the patient's ECG in accordance with procedures in Chapter 2 if your place of work has an ECG machine. Do not worry if you cannot interpret the ECG results as modern automated equipment provides an interpretation for you. These modern ECG machines tend to over-diagnose the problem of heart attack but it is better to be safe than sorry.

Once we suspect or can confirm the diagnosis of myocardial infarction, as in George's case, we normally start treatment to restore blood flow to the coronary arteries. The treatment of myocardial infarction, like any other treatment, should take into account your patient's individual needs and preferences. In partnership with your patient, you should allow the patient the opportunity to make informed decisions about care and treatment. In some instances, your patient may lack capacity to decide, in which case you should let the Mental Capacity Act 2005 guide you. In George's case, you could involve his wife in the decision-making process if George consents.

We mainly use a cocktail of medicines that include thrombolytics, beta-blockers, angiotensin-converting enzyme (ACE) inhibitors, anticoagulants and anticlotting medicines. In addition to these medicines, we can apply a surgical procedure we call angioplasty to remedy myocardial infarction.

Thrombolytic medicines

Thrombolytics or clot busters are medicines we use to dissolve blood clots that block the coronary arteries. These drugs assume a central role in the therapy of acute and chronic coronary artery disease. They work best when we give them within several hours (up to 18 hours) of the onset of a myocardial infarction (Collins *et al.* 1997). In addition, they increase a person's chances of surviving a myocardial infarction or heart attack and of being alive for at least 12 years after the first attack (French *et al.* 1999). All thrombolytic medicines are equally effective and work for all types of heart attacks (Collins *et al.* 1997). Some common examples of thrombolytic medicines are alteplase, reteplase, streptokinase and tenecteplase. For details of dosages and side-effect management of these medicines, please consult a textbook on medicines management.

Beta-blockers

Beta-blockers are a class of medicines that work by blocking the effects of the hormone adrenaline. When taken, these medicines block the adrenaline receptors (β-adrenergic), making the heart beat more slowly and with less force, thereby reducing blood pressure and the heart's workload. We also use beta-blockers to relieve chest pain and discomfort. Some common beta-blockers include acebutolol, atenolol, bisoprolol, metoprolol and propranolol. For their management, please consult a book on medicines management.

ACE inhibitors

ACE inhibitors are a class of medicines that have common use in treating high blood pressure (hypertension). They work by reducing the activity of the hormone angiotensin, which constricts blood vessels and this leads to widening (dilation) of blood vessels. The widening of blood vessels will result in the reduction of blood pressure. The reduction in blood pressure reduces the heart work rate and slows down kidney disease progression that is due to high blood pressure or diabetes.

ACE inhibitors include medicines such as ramipril, captopril, enalapril, fosinopril, lisinopril and quinapril. These medicines are generally effective in the control of blood pressure. A Cochrane review of 92 trials that assessed the effectiveness of 14 different ACE inhibitors concluded that all ACE inhibitors are equally effective (Heran *et al.* 2009).

Anticoagulants

Blood clots that impede normal vascular blood flow are an aggregation of red blood cells, platelets, fibrin and white blood cells. To overcome the problem, we use anticoagulants to stop these components from aggregating and forming a clot and to prevent existing blood clots from getting bigger. We sometimes refer to anticoagulants as 'blood thinners'. The term blood thinner can be misleading, as some anticoagulants actually work by increasing the time it takes for blood to clot. Common anticoagulants are warfarin, heparin and the newer anticoagulants such as dabigatran, rivaroxaban and apixaban. The newer anticoagulants are equally effective (Fox *et al.* 2012). For the safe management of these medicines, please consult a book on medicines management.

Tertiary prevention of cardiovascular disease

In tertiary prevention, we aim to prevent further deterioration of a disease and rehabilitate the individual. In doing so, we aim to return the patient to a status of maximum usefulness with a minimum risk of recurrence of a physical or mental disorder. You should therefore discuss options for preventing further illness episodes with your patient. Tertiary prevention strategies of CHD usually involve lifestyle changes that include exercise and dietary changes. To ensure that your patient recovers optimally from CHD, you should work closely with the patient's GP, who may refer the patient for cardiac rehabilitation. Patients with mental health problems generally experience problems in accessing appropriate healthcare and therefore you should support and guide where appropriate in this endeavour. Additionally, you should take into account your patient's wider health and social needs; this may involve you assisting in identifying and addressing economic, welfare rights, housing or social support issues. Social needs are usually areas of concern for many patients with mental health problems.

Cardiac rehabilitation

Cardiac rehabilitation is a programme that helps people with cardiovascular problems to improve their health and well-being. It includes exercise training, education, healthy living and counselling to reduce stress and help the person to return to an active life. Cardiac rehabilitation programmes should be culturally sensitive and should be able to cater to the needs of your patient. As mentioned earlier, dietary changes are important in secondary prevention

Dietary changes

Using health-promoting strategies outlined in Chapter 3, you should work with your patient with a view to making dietary changes. You should discuss the unsuitability of certain foods or supplements rich in beta-carotene. These foods include sweet potatoes, kale, carrots, turnips, dried herbs and butternut squash. In a meta-analysis with 138,113 participants, beta-carotene led to a statistically significant increase in all-cause mortality and cardiovascular death. The investigators concluded that patients should be 'actively discouraged' from taking supplements that contain beta-carotene. They called their findings 'especially concerning' because beta-carotene doses are a common constituent in over-the-counter vitamin supplements and multivitamin supplements that have widespread usage (Vivekananthan *et al.* 2003). The same meta-analytic study found that antioxidant supplements such as vitamin E or C, or folic acid do not play any useful role in reducing cardiovascular risk.

You should also discuss with your patient the advantages of consuming food rich in omega fatty acids. The National Institute for Health and Care Excellence (NICE) guidelines suggest people should eat at least 7 grams of omega-3 fatty acids per week from two to four portions of oily fish (NICE 2007a). Foods rich in omega-3 fatty acids are flaxseed, walnuts, soybeans and fish like salmon, sardines and halibut. Among many functions, omega-3 fatty acids keep our blood from clotting excessively and lower the amount of fats such as LDL-C and triglycerides in our blood. They also decrease platelet aggregation, therefore prevent excessive blood clotting. More importantly, the omega-3 fatty acids may reduce the risk of obesity and improve the body's ability to respond to insulin by stimulating the secretion of leptin, a hormone that helps regulate food intake, body weight and metabolism. However, some recent empirical evidence challenges the effectiveness of omega-3 fatty acids in the secondary prevention of CVD (Bosch *et al.* 2012; Kwak *et al.* 2012). The importance of omega-3 fatty acid is discussed in more detail in Chapter 9.

In addition to omega-3 fatty acids, you should discuss and highlight the importance of eating a Mediterranean-style diet (see Chapter 9). In advising patients about diet, tailor this around the patient's needs and preferences. These should take into account your patient's financial resources, culture, ethnicity or religion. Alcohol consumption has a deleterious effect on the cardiovascular system and therefore you should discuss this if your patient drinks alcohol. In any event, it is advisable not to drink more than 21 units a week for men and 14 units per week for women.

Smoking cessation

There is a strong association between smoking cessation and a substantial reduction in risk of all-cause mortality among patients with CHD. A Cochrane review of 20 studies found a reduction of 36% in relative risk of death for those who quit smoking compared to those who continued to smoke. The review also found a reduction in non-fatal myocardial infarction in those who stopped smoking (Critchley and Capewell 2004). This risk reduction is consistent, irrespective of differences between the studies in terms of index cardiac events, age, sex, country and period. A disproportionately high number of patients with serious mental illness smoke and therefore, by applying motivational interviewing principles discussed in Chapter 3, you can explore the possibility of your patient giving up smoking. Further, you may offer support and advice to all patients who express a desire to quit smoking and, in some cases, referral to some intensive support service such as the NHS Stop Smoking Services is in order. In some cases, it may be appropriate for the patient to use pharmacological smoking cessation aids. Evidence-based guidelines recommend nicotine replacement therapy, bupropion SR, and varenicline as effective alternatives for smoking cessation therapy, especially in combination with behavioural interventions (see Chapter 7).

Regular physical activity

Exercise-based cardiac rehabilitation aims to restore patients with heart disease to health. A Cochrane systematic review that analysed 47 studies with a total patient sample of 10,794 patients found that exercise-based cardiac rehabilitation is effective in reducing cardiovascular mortality and hospital admissions (Heran *et al.* 2011). In this respect, it is important to advise patients to take up exercise to increase cardiac capacity. Physical activity of 20–30 minutes a day to the point of slight breathlessness is particularly effective. Patients who have difficulties in achieving this goal can increase their activity in a gradual, systematic way, aiming to increase their exercise capacity. They should start at a level that is comfortable, and increase the duration and intensity of activity as they gain fitness. Advice on physical activity should involve a discussion about current and past activity levels and preferences. To enhance the benefit of exercise you may need to refer your patient to a suitability qualified professional (see Chapter 9).

Heart failure

Heart failure is a condition where the heart cannot pump enough blood to meet the body's needs. The condition can affect the right side or, more commonly, both sides of the heart. Right-side heart failure occurs when the heart cannot pump enough blood to the lungs for oxygenation. This type of heart failure may cause fluid to build up in the feet, ankles, legs, liver, abdomen and the veins in the neck. Left-side heart failure occurs when the heart cannot pump enough oxygen-rich blood to the rest of the body. Right-side and left-side heart failure also may cause shortness of breath and fatigue. Before you read further, please take part in the activity below.

Activity 4.3 *Critical thinking*

May is 41 years old and suffers from depression and has recently been diagnosed with breast cancer. She has been treated with chemotherapy drugs called anthracyclines for 9 months. Although she has no known heart problems, her oncologist referred her to a cardiologist. Can you suggest why she has been referred to a cardiologist even though she has no known cardiac problems?

Any condition that damages or overworks the heart muscle can cause heart failure. Over time, the heart weakens because it is not able to fill or pump blood as well as it should and this results in the release of certain proteins and substances into the blood. These proteins and substances have a toxic effect on the blood and worsen heart failure.

As we discussed earlier, the most common causes of heart failure are CHD, high blood pressure and diabetes.

Heart failure is more common in:

- people who are 65 years old or older, as ageing can weaken the heart muscle. Older people with mental health problems may have had the condition for many years without detection;

- people with darker skin and particularly those of African Caribbean, Indian, Pakistani or Bangladeshi background are more likely to have heart failure in comparison to people of other races. They are also more likely to have heart failure symptoms and die at a younger age;

- obese people, because excess weight puts a strain on the heart and increases the risk of developing type 2 diabetes, which increases the risk for heart failure (see Chapter 5);

- men, who have a higher rate of heart failure than women.

Signs and symptoms of heart failure

Shortness of breath or trouble breathing
Fatigue (tiredness)
Swelling in the ankles, feet, legs, abdomen and veins in the neck. Fluid build-up from heart failure also causes weight gain, frequent urination and a cough that is worse at night and when the person is lying down. This cough may be a sign of acute pulmonary oedema, a condition where there is too much fluid building up in a person's lungs. Quite often, we treat this condition as a medical emergency
High and weak pulse

Table 4.1: Signs and symptoms of heart failure

The symptoms listed in Table 4.1 are mainly due to the accumulation of fluid in the body. A person may feel tired and short of breath at the start of heart failure. This is particularly noticeable after routine physical effort such as climbing up the stairs or doing light jogging. With time, the heart gets weaker and the symptoms deteriorate. At this stage, a person may feel tired and short of breath after performing very light activities like getting dressed or walking across the room. In some situations, people may have shortness of breath while lying flat. Because people with serious mental illness such as depression and schizophrenia do not readily come forward and tell you their symptoms, you need to be proactive in eliciting symptoms.

Treatment of heart failure

The prognosis for those with heart failure is generally poor. In this respect, the treatment of heart failure aims to treat the condition's underlying cause, such as CVD, high blood pressure or diabetes. The other aspect of treatment of heart failure is to reduce symptoms and stop the heart failure from deteriorating. The final part of treatment should aim to increase the individual's lifespan and quality of life. In this respect, treatment will normally include lifestyle changes, medicines and ongoing care.

In terms of pharmacological treatment, ACE inhibitors and beta-blockers are the treatment of choice if the patient is suffering from left ventricular failure. In addition to ACE inhibitors, diuretics may help the patient to reduce fluid build-up in the lungs and swelling in the feet and ankles. However, the use of diuretics in people with heart failure can be problematic, because people with heart failure tend to retain fluid and will require diuretics to help excrete excess fluid. If the patient then loses too much fluid, potassium is also lost. Potassium plays a major role in the electrical stimulation of cells such as nerve and muscle cells. Therefore, lack of potassium can cause very rapid heart rhythms that can lead to sudden death. In this respect, monitoring the balance between fluid retention and potassium loss is critical for heart failure patients. One way of achieving this is the use of potassium-sparing diuretics like aldosterone antagonists. These medicines include spironolactone and eplerenone and they trigger the body to get rid of salt and water through urine. However, aldosterone antagonists do not promote the secretion of potassium into the urine; thus, they spare potassium and do not lose it as much as other diuretics do.

Another effective way of treating heart failure is the use of medicines that relax blood vessels such as isosorbide dinitrate or hydralazine hydrochloride. Of particular interest is the finding in the USA that this medicinal combination can reduce the risk of death in African Americans (Seguin *et al.* 2008). However, we need to find out more about whether this medicine will benefit other racial groups.

In addition to medicines, you work with patients with a view to making changes to their lifestyle. These lifestyle changes include diet and exercise. Before you read further, please take part in the activity below.

Activity 4.4

John, a 54-year-old male who suffers from depression, was also diagnosed with congestive cardiac failure 2 years ago and he takes furosemide. You have noticed recently that John has developed poor appetite, nausea, drowsiness and feelings of apprehension, fatigue, muscle pain and weakness in the legs. What may be your concerns regarding John?

Diet and exercise

It is important to discuss the possibility of following a healthy diet as part of managing heart failure. An inappropriate diet can lead to worsening of the condition and therefore, it is appropriate to work closely with other members of the multidisciplinary team like the dietician. A healthy diet may include fresh vegetables and fruits, whole grains and fat-free or low-fat dairy products. In addition, the diet can include protein foods, such as lean meats, eggs, seafood, nuts, seeds, beans, peas and poultry without skin (see Chapter 9).

As we discussed earlier, it is necessary to advise the patient regarding the role of potassium. As with insufficient potassium, excess potassium can be harmful. Potassium-rich foods that include potato skins, white beans, greens, bananas, mushrooms, avocados and salmon should be eaten sparingly. You should also discuss the role of a low-sodium and low-saturated-fat diet. Excess sodium can cause excess fluid to build up in the body, therefore making the heart condition worse. *Trans*-fatty acids and saturated fat can increase blood cholesterol levels which, as discussed previously, are a risk factor for heart disease.

Patients with heart failure tend to be intolerant of exercise, as they tend to experience early fatigue and shortness of breath. These symptoms influence the patient's ability to perform activities of daily living, reducing the patient's capacity to participate meaningfully. However, available evidence overwhelmingly suggests that exercise for people with heart failure is safe and provides substantial physiological and psychological benefits (Adsett *et al.* 2013). As such, we now consider exercise as part of the non-pharmacological management of patients with heart failure. Aerobic training is particularly useful in improving the physiological components of aerobic metabolism such as improvement in peak oxygen uptake. We will discuss the importance of exercise in Chapter 9.

Cerebrovascular accident

Case study

Christine is a 47-year-old woman who suffers from depression and anxiety. A few years ago, she was diagnosed with type 2 diabetes but she had not been closely monitoring her blood sugar levels, most likely due to her mental health. As a result, her diabetes has been poorly controlled and she was diagnosed with hypertension a year ago. Two weeks ago, Christine suffered a moderate cerebrovascular accident (CVA). Prior to the stroke, she functioned independently.

The World Health Organization defines CVA or stroke as *a clinical syndrome consisting of rapidly developing clinical signs of focal (or global in case of coma) disturbance of cerebral function lasting more than 24 hours or leading to death with no apparent cause other than a vascular origin* (WHO 2014c). Stroke is a major health problem in the UK and each year, approximately 110,000 people such as Christine have a first or recurrent stroke. In mental health, the prevalence and incidence of stroke are nearly twice as much compared to the general population, particularly for stroke and mental health conditions such as depression (Pan *et al.* 2011) and schizophrenia (Tsai *et al.* 2012). This is because most of the risk factors for stroke are present in abundance in people with mental health problems. Such risk factors include obesity, smoking, alcohol consumption and diabetes, as in the case of Christine.

Most strokes happen when a blood clot blocks one of the arteries that carry blood to the brain in a similar manner that causes cardiac ischaemia. We sometimes refer to the process of blockage of brain arteries by a blood clot as ischaemic stroke. Approximately 80% of strokes happen this way. Another cause of stroke is haemorrhagic stroke, due to the rupture of an artery within the brain triggering an intracerebral haemorrhage (15% of strokes).

Risk factors

The risk factors for the development of stroke are similar to those of any CVD and we have discussed these earlier. Briefly, these risk factors include hypertension, smoking, diabetes, alcohol intake and high cholesterol.

Symptoms of a stroke

Strokes usually happen suddenly and no two strokes are the same, as people can be affected in quite different ways. How the stroke happens depends in part on the location of brain where the damage is. This is because different parts of the brain control different functions, such as speaking, memory, swallowing and moving. The most common signs of a stroke are:

- weakness down one side of the body, ranging from numbness to paralysis that can affect the arm and leg;
- weakness down one side of the face, causing the mouth to droop;
- speech may be difficult or become difficult to understand;
- swallowing may be affected;
- loss of muscle coordination or balance;
- brief loss of vision;
- severe headache;
- confusion.

People who have had a severe stroke may lose consciousness and unfortunately, the likelihood of such patients making a good recovery is poor.

The face–arm–speech test (FAST)

The UK Stroke Association (2006) says there are three simple checks that can help you to recognise whether someone has had a stroke or mini-stroke. This simple test checks the individual's face, arm and speech and when you test for these symptoms and they are present, you call the ambulance (by dialling 999) straight away. We know this simple test by the acronym FAST:

- Facial weakness: can the person smile? Has the mouth or eye drooped?

- Arm weakness: can the person raise both arms?

- Speech problems: can the person speak clearly and understand you?

- Time to call ambulance: if a person shows any of these symptoms, even if the symptoms go away, call an ambulance and get the person to the hospital immediately. Make a note of the time so you know when the first symptoms appeared.

Treatment of stroke

The first thing in the treatment of a stroke is to ascertain what type of stroke the patient has had and we do this using a scan. If a blood clot is the cause, we use 'clot-busting' medication to dissolve the clot, but you must give this within 3 hours of the stroke. You may give anti-clotting medication such as aspirin to stop the stroke from getting worse. If the stroke is due to haemorrhage, you do not give anti-clotting medication as this medicine makes the bleeding worse. You should ensure you perform key neurological tests and key functions such as swallowing and movement. In addition, monitor oxygen, glucose and blood pressure levels if possible.

During the first few days after a stroke, you should focus on ensuring that your patient receives sufficient fluids and nutrition. The next stage should involve the services of other health professionals, including physiotherapists, speech therapists, occupational therapists, nurses and doctors.

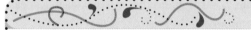

Chapter summary

Cardiovascular disorders rank first as the world leading cause of mortality and this problem compounds significantly in people with mental health problems. In particular, people with depression, schizophrenia and anxiety are at an increased risk of developing cardiovascular problems because risk factors for the disease are abundant in this population. These risk factors are obesity, hypertension, diabetes, sedentary lifestyle, smoking and alcohol use. These factors promote the development of atherosclerosis, a key substance in cardiovascular disorder. Treatment and management of cardiovascular disorders mainly centre on ameliorating risk factors. Anti-clotting agents, ACE inhibitors and antihypertensives are among some of the pharmacological approaches we use to manage this condition.

Activities: brief outline of answers

Activity 4.1

Sleep disorders such as **apnoea** can raise the risk for hypertension, diabetes, and even a heart attack or stroke. Sleep disorders are very common in people with mental health problems.

Activity 4.2

You could encourage patients to eat certain foods that help to raise HDL-C in the body, such as raw onions, whole grain, oats, oat bran, brown rice, citrus fruits, grapes, apples, legumes and lentils. You should encourage patients to exercise for at least 20 minutes three times a week as this increases HDL-C.

Activity 4.3

Antracyclines elevate the risk of heart failure.

Activity 4.4

Quite possibly, John is experiencing symptoms of potassium depletion (hypokalaemia). You need to alert the doctor as soon as possible. You may wish to take an ECG while you are waiting for the doctor to arrive. ECG changes you might see include a decrease in the T-wave amplitude, ST-segment depression and T-wave inversions.

Further reading

Nash M (2009) *Physical Health and Well Being in Mental Health Nursing: Clinical skills for practice.* Maidenhead, Berkshire: Open University.

Useful websites

http://www.patient.co.uk/doctor/stroke-prevention

This website is specifically geared for patients with cardiovascular problems and it offers useful advice.

http://www.bhf.org.uk/#&panel1-2

This is a useful website that explains CVD and its management in lay language.

Chapter 5
Metabolic syndrome and diabetes mellitus

NMC Standards for Pre-registration Nursing Education

This chapter will address the following competencies:

Domain 1: Professional values

Generic standard for competence

All nurses must act first and foremost to care for and safeguard the public. They must practise autonomously and be responsible and accountable for safe, compassionate, person-centred, evidence-based nursing that respects and maintains dignity and human rights. They must show professionalism, integrity, and work within recognised professional, ethical and legal frameworks. They must work in partnership with other health and social care professionals and agencies, service users, their carers and families in all settings, including the community, ensuring that decisions about care are shared.

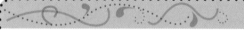

NMC Essential Skills Clusters

This chapter will address the following ESCs:

1. As partners in the care process, people can trust a newly registered graduate nurse to provide collaborative care based on the highest standards, knowledge and competence.
9. People can trust the newly registered graduate nurse to treat them as partners and work with them to make a holistic and systematic assessment of their needs; to develop a personalised plan that is based on mutual understanding and respect for their individual situation promoting health and well-being, minimising risk of harm and promoting their safety at all times.

Chapter aims

By the end of the chapter, you should be able to:

- understand and describe metabolic syndrome;
- discuss the risk factors associated with metabolic syndrome and diabetes;
- discuss primary, secondary and tertiary interventions for metabolic syndrome and diabetes.

Introduction

During your clinical practice you will come across some people who are overweight and this state may be causing them considerable problems. Possibly, they may be suffering from a metabolic syndrome. Metabolic syndrome is a collection of conditions or risk factors for heart disease, diabetes and stroke. We also know this condition as syndrome X, insulin resistance syndrome, dysmetabolic syndrome or Reaven's syndrome.

This condition is quite common and affects about 25% of adults in Europe and Latin America. Some racial and ethnic groups are at higher risk of this condition than others. In the USA, Mexican Americans have the highest rate of metabolic syndrome, followed by Caucasians and African Americans. The rate of metabolic syndrome is rising in developing countries in East Asia. Metabolic syndrome is also common in people who have a sibling or parent with diabetes and there is evidence of a genetic basis for the condition (Groop 2000). Other groups at risk are women who have a history of polycystic ovarian disease, and people with mental health problems who are significantly at increased risk of metabolic syndrome in comparison to the general population. In general, the prevalence of metabolic syndrome increases with age, and about 40% of people over the age of 60 years have the condition.

Concept summary

For a diagnosis of metabolic syndrome, at least three of the following conditions ought to be present:

1. an increase in abdominal fat, especially a waist circumference of 88 cm (35 inches) or more in women and 102 cm (40 inches) or more in men. Excess fat in the stomach area is a greater risk factor for heart disease than excess fat in other parts of the body;
2. a high blood level of triglycerides;
3. a low high-density lipoprotein cholesterol (HDL-C) level or 'good' cholesterol (see Chapter 4). An HDL-C level of less than 1.3 mmol/L for women and less than 1.0 mmol/L for men is a metabolic risk factor;
4. high blood pressure of 130/85 mmHg or more;
5. high fasting blood glucose level of 2.8 mmol/L or above.

The bulk of evidence in support of the prevalence of metabolic syndrome in mental health comes from patients with schizophrenia or depression and, to a lesser extent, from patients with bipolar disorder (Haupt and Newcomer 2002). From a worldwide perspective, increase in calorie intake and sedentary lifestyles are the factors responsible for the development of metabolic syndrome (Papanastasiou 2012). These factors are very common in people with mental health problems (see Chapter 1). Metabolic syndrome is more likely in people taking second-generation antipsychotics than first-generation antipsychotics, and in those on **polypharmacy** rather than **monopharmacy**. It is also more likely in those taking low-potency antipsychotics in comparison to high-potency antipsychotics. For individual antipsychotics, clozapine and olanzapine are more likely to cause higher metabolic syndrome rates than other antipsychotics. Metabolic syndrome can also be found in people who are treatment-naïve. In an influential study, the Clinical Antipsychotic Trials of Intervention Effectiveness (CATIE) found that approximately one-third of patients met the criteria for metabolic syndrome at treatment initiation (Meyer *et al.* 2008).

This chapter will discuss the role of obesity and its link to type 2 diabetes before addressing symptoms and interventions of type 2 diabetes in more detail. First, we will look at the link between obesity and mental health.

Prevalence of obesity

Case study

*Yvette is a 52-year-old woman who has suffered from depression for the past 9 years and her treatment is clomipramine. For the past 6 months, she has noticed a marked decrease in her energy level, particularly in the afternoons. She has gained a great deal of weight over the years; her body mass index (BMI) is now 32 kg/m² and most of her weight is around the abdominal area. She states that every time she tries to cut down on her eating she has symptoms of shakiness, **diaphoresis** and increased hunger. She does not follow any specific diet and her care coordinator has repeatedly advised her to lose weight and exercise to improve her health status. However, she complains that the pain in her knees and ankles makes it difficult to do any exercise.*

In common parlance, obesity may simply mean an increased body weight caused by excessive accumulation of fat. It is a serious and complex health concern that confronts the developed world. In the UK, obesity has increased dramatically over the past 25 years, with 25% of all adults being obese. If current trends continue, 90% of adults in the UK could be obese by 2050; this is likely to have important ramifications for the NHS and the economy. At a BMI of 32 kg/m², we can consider Yvette to be obese and current estimates are that obesity directly costs the NHS £4.2 billion a year. The indirect costs of the condition to the economy approximate to £16 billion a year.

Obesity shortens life, and is a risk factor for various diseases, like cardiovascular diseases, diabetes and cancer. Of all the associated comorbidities, type 2 diabetes shows the strongest link with obesity. Specifically, abdominal/visceral obesity, as in Yvette's case, is a known risk factor for the development of type 2 diabetes mellitus (also known as 'insulin-resistant' or 'adult-onset' diabetes). The longer an individual remains obese, the higher the person's risk level of developing type 2 diabetes mellitus.

Type 2 diabetes and mental health

Approximately 40 million people die as a direct result of complications of diabetes a year and this figure accounts for 9% of all global deaths. More than 80% of people dying from diabetes are from low- and middle-income countries. According to the World Health Organization (WHO), the number of people with diabetes worldwide will increase to at least 300 million by

2025 and it will be the seventh leading cause of death by 2030 (WHO 2011a). Of the people diagnosed with type 2 diabetes, about 80–90% are also obese. According to the Centers for Disease Control in the USA (Khan *et al.* 2009), we are eating ourselves into a diabetes epidemic. The International Diabetes Foundation states that, *Diabetes and obesity are the biggest public health challenges of the 21st century.* People with mental health problems are more likely to have metabolic syndrome and by extension are at elevated risk for developing type 2 diabetes. In particular, people with schizophrenia are inherently at risk from developing type 2 diabetes even in the absence of risk factors. In 1899, the psychiatrist Henry Maudsley observed that:

> *Diabetes is a disease which often shows itself in families in which insanity prevails: whether one disease predisposes in any way to the other or not, or whether they are independent outcomes of a common neurosis, they are certainly found to run side by side, or alternately with one another more often than can be accounted for by accidental coincidence or sequence.*

Recent epidemiological studies support this early observation by Henry Maudsley. For example, a recent study found that the incidence of type 2 diabetes in people with schizophrenia was significantly higher than in those without schizophrenia (Schoepf *et al.* 2012). Other investigators have found that the prevalence of diabetes in people with schizophrenia is 16–25% higher than in the general population (Yogaratnam *et al.* 2013). Further, accumulating genetic evidence supports the view that the genes responsible for schizophrenia are also responsible for type 2 diabetes (Liu *et al.* 2013). Similarly, diabetes appears inherent in those with depression.

More than 300 years ago Dr Thomas Willis, a British physician, observed a relationship between diabetes and depression and suggested that diabetes was the result of *sadness or long sorrow* (Willis 1971). A meta-analysis of 42 published studies found that the prevalence of major depression in people with diabetes was 11%. Other authors suggest that, in comparison to those who do not suffer from diabetes, people with type 2 diabetes are at least one-and-a-half times more likely to suffer from depression (Mezuk *et al.* 2008).

Apart from the inherent relationship, we attribute much of this elevated risk to the use of psychotropic medication which causes metabolic abnormalities in people with mental health problems. In the treatment of schizophrenia, the risk for the development of metabolic abnormalities that leads to type 2 diabetes mellitus is highest with clozapine and olanzapine. With regard to the treatment of depression, antidepressants with noradrenergic activity such as tricyclics, like imipramine, and serotonin–noradrenaline reuptake inhibitors like venlafaxine have the highest potential to cause metabolic abnormalities. Further, evidence suggests that people with type 2 diabetes mellitus and depression have significantly higher **proinflammatory markers** (Howren *et al.* 2009) in comparison to those with diabetes but who are not depressed. Similarly, those with type 2 diabetes mellitus and depression show significantly higher levels of the proinflammatory protein C-reactive protein (Doyle *et al.* 2013). These findings suggest that inflammation is a shared pathophysiological mechanism in both type 2 diabetes and depression.

In addition, some people have difficulties in coping with diabetes and this may contribute to the development of a mental health problem. For example, a recent study that examined the prevalence of mental health disorders in people with diabetes found that, of the 200 participants, 43% had at least one mental health disorder. The most common disorders were generalised anxiety disorder (21%), dysthymia (15%), social phobia (7%), current depression (5.5%) and lifelong depression (3.5%), panic disorder (2.5%) and risk of suicide (2%) (Maia *et al.* 2012). If not controlled, diabetes can lead to a number of complications.

Before an individual develops diabetes, a condition we call pre-diabetes or insulin resistance predates it. To understand insulin resistance, we need to look at the role that insulin plays in the regulation of glucose in the blood.

Role of insulin and glucagon

The key organ in the metabolism of glucose is the pancreas, which lies behind the stomach (Figure 5.1). The function of the pancreas is twofold: it produces pancreatic juice, a digestive enzyme that breaks down ingested food (fats and proteins); and it produces hormones to regulate bodily functions. The two main pancreatic hormones that regulate blood glucose are insulin and glucagon.

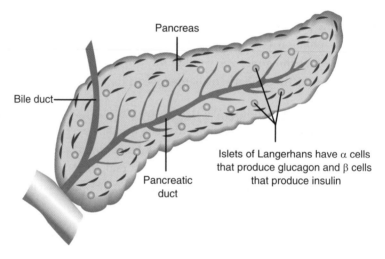

Figure 5.1: The pancreas, showing the islets of Langerhans

When we eat carbohydrates, they are broken down in the digestive system before being absorbed into the blood as glucose. The absorption temporarily raises blood glucose levels above the normal level, which can be as high as 8 mmol/L soon after meals. Before you read further, please take part in the activity below.

Activity 5.1 — *Critical thinking*

Peter, a patient who suffers from schizophrenia and has type 2 diabetes mellitus, has his blood sugar monitored before meals. However, a nurse took blood glucose levels about 10 minutes after breakfast. What are your concerns about the reading?

There are outline answers to all the activities at the end of the chapter.

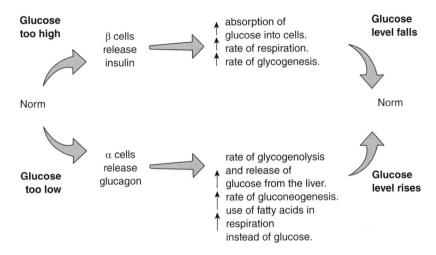

Figure 5.2: Insulin–glucagon cycle

To bring the blood glucose levels to within normal limits, pancreatic beta cells produce insulin and excrete it into the blood stream. The insulin helps body cells use glucose for metabolism. It acts like a key that opens up cell doors to allow glucose from the blood to enter into the cells. Insulin also induces the liver to convert and store excess glucose as glycogen. Both these actions result in blood glucose levels falling to normal levels in individuals who have no diabetes. If blood glucose levels fall below normal, as in the case of intensive physical exercise or between meals, the alpha cells of the pancreas secrete the hormone glucagon. Glucagon helps to convert the stored glycogen in the liver back to glucose, increasing the glucose levels in the blood (Figure 5.2).

In people with type 2 diabetes, the process of regulating blood glucose is defective. First, the beta cells of the pancreas may not produce enough insulin to convert excess glucose to glycogen or to facilitate more glucose to enter the cells for metabolism.

In either case, blood glucose levels will rise to above normal levels, producing hyperglycaemia. Second, the alpha cells of the pancreas may not produce enough glucagon hormone to convert glycogen back to glucose, and this results in blood glucose levels falling below normal, producing **hypoglycaemia**. Prior to the onset of diabetes, the body cells resist the effects of insulin, a condition we call insulin resistance.

Insulin resistance

As we discussed earlier, one of insulin's jobs is to facilitate glucose entry into cells for metabolism. However, this process is not straightforward in insulin resistance. This is because there is a reduction in the cells' ability to respond to insulin's facilitation. Put differently, when the cell doors do not open when insulin knocks, we call this insulin resistance. To compensate for this deficiency, the beta cells of the pancreas respond by producing more insulin to produce an effect. In other words, the insulin knocks on the door even louder to produce an effect. If this overproduction of insulin continues, it results in a condition we call **hyperinsulinaemia**, which means 'too much insulin in the blood'. Hyperinsulinaemia causes other problems, including making it more difficult for the body to use stored fat for energy. It also causes weight gain, particularly abdominal

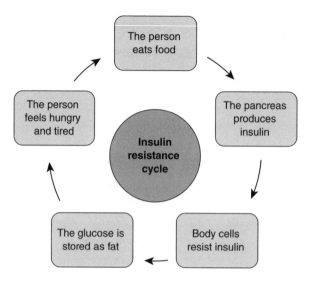

Figure 5.3: The insulin resistance cycle

obesity, high blood pressure, high triglycerides and low HDL-C. These conditions are part of metabolic syndrome and insulin resistance is integral to this condition.

There has been much debate regarding the cause of insulin resistance but we now believe obesity plays a key part in the process. We consider obesity a low-grade inflammatory condition of the white fat tissues which results in these tissues overproducing a wide range of substances that cause inflammation (proinflammatory), such as tumour necrosis factor-alpha and interleukin-6 (Howren *et al.* 2009). These inflammatory markers interfere with insulin's role in aiding glucose metabolism (Bastard *et al.* 2006). This prompts the pancreas to secrete more and more insulin and eventually, blood glucose levels rise out of control and the person develops type 2 diabetes mellitus (Figure 5.3).

Before you proceed further, please take part in the next activity.

Activity 5.2

In a group or individually, find out which psychotropic medications are least likely to cause diabetes.

Signs and symptoms of diabetes mellitus

Symptoms of type 1 and type 2 diabetes mellitus may manifest in several ways and, in spite of differences, the warning signs of diabetes tend to overlap. For the most part, symptoms are usually much less severe in type 2 than in type 1 diabetes. For this reason, some people can go for years without even knowing they have the condition. However, below is a summary of the signs and symptoms of type 2 diabetes mellitus which you need to look out for.

Frequent urination

This is a common symptom of type 2 diabetes mellitus and it occurs when there is too much glucose in the blood. If insulin is non-existent or ineffective, the kidneys cannot filter glucose back to the blood. They become overwhelmed and, to compensate for this, they try to draw extra water out of the blood to dilute the glucose. This keeps the bladder full and causes frequent urination.

Excessive thirst

If an individual is drinking more than usual, it could be a sign of type 2 diabetes mellitus, particularly if excessive thirst accompanies frequent urination. The excessive thirst is due to the body drawing excess water from the blood and therefore filling the bladder more. The individual then suffers dehydration and as a result, drinks more to replenish the lost water. Be aware that some psychotropic medications such as tricyclic antidepressants and low-potency antipsychotics also cause excessive thirst.

Weight loss

As a symptom, weight loss is more apparent in those with type 1 diabetes and this is because the pancreas stops making insulin. This may be because of a viral attack on the insulin-producing cells or this may be due to an autoimmune response that attacks the insulin-producing cells (beta cells). This results in the body lacking an energy source and it responds by breaking fat and protein from muscle to obtain energy. Because type 2 diabetes mellitus occurs insidiously and proportionately to insulin resistance, weight loss is not as noticeable.

Tiredness

After eating, glucose enters the blood stream but if there is no insulin, the glucose is unable to enter the cells or to be stored as glycogen in the liver (Figure 5.3). Consequently, the body cells become energy-deficient and the individual feels tired. This symptom overlaps with side effects of some low-potency antipsychotics such as olanzapine and tricyclic antidepressants such as imipramine. Furthermore, depressive and negative symptoms can overlap with tiredness from glucose dysregulation.

Tingling sensation or numbness in extremities

We call this symptom neuropathy and it is due to consistently high blood glucose which damages the nervous system. Specifically, it damages body extremities. The tingling sensation and numbness of the extremities will often diminish with an improvement in blood glucose regulation.

Blurred vision

High blood glucose causes the lens of the eye to swell, causing blurry vision. When the blood glucose level goes back to normal, the blurry vision usually disappears. This symptom overlaps with psychotropic-induced blurry vision.

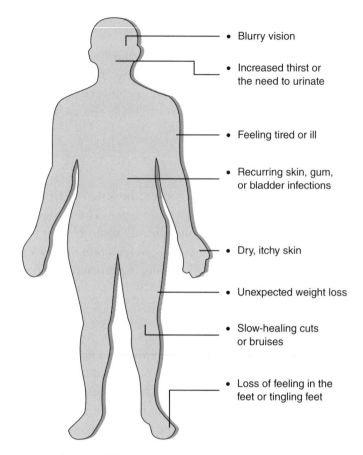

- Blurry vision
- Increased thirst or the need to urinate
- Feeling tired or ill
- Recurring skin, gum, or bladder infections
- Dry, itchy skin
- Unexpected weight loss
- Slow-healing cuts or bruises
- Loss of feeling in the feet or tingling feet

Figure 5.4: Symptoms and signs of diabetes

Frequent infections

Because diabetes injures the immune system, individuals are at an elevated risk of infections. Control of blood glucose will result in improvement of the immune system and therefore lessen the chances of contracting an infection.

Increased hunger

We call this condition polyphagia and this is because, when blood glucose levels are high, the body's tissues are not able to take up the glucose and use it correctly as energy. This is because the body cells are resistant to insulin (Figure 5.3). Polyphagia, along with polyuria and polydipsia, tends to be much milder in type 2 diabetes mellitus than in type 1 diabetes.

Slow-healing wounds

Slow-healing wounds are usually due to poor blood circulation. This is why diabetes is the leading cause of lower-extremity amputations.

Lack of interest and concentration

This symptom overlaps with the lack of interest and poor concentration we see in people with negative symptoms of schizophrenia and those with depression.

Vomiting and stomach pain

These gastrointestinal symptoms are more common in patients with diabetes and often reflect diabetic gastrointestinal autonomic neuropathy. Before you read further, please take part in the activity below.

Activity 5.3 — *Critical thinking*

Study Figure 5.4. Make a list of the symptoms of diabetes that overlap with mental health symptoms and psychotropic side effects.

Screening test for diabetes

Early screening for diabetes reduces the risk of complications and loss of life-years. We use two main methods to screen type 2 diabetes mellitus – fasting blood sugar and oral glucose tolerance test (OGTT) – and nurses play an important role in both these tests.

Fasting blood sugar

We use the fasting blood sugar test to screen for a pre-diabetic condition. In this test, the patient cannot eat or drink anything except water for a period of up to 10 hours before the test. You should discourage the patient from taking any caffeine or caffeine product, as this distorts the results of the test. Continually remind those patients with cognitive symptoms about the need not to eat during the period before the test. Most people prefer to go for the test first thing in the morning after fasting all night. After fasting, the normal blood glucose levels should be within the range of 4–7 mmol/L. If fasting blood glucose levels reach or exceed 7 mmol/L, then this is a cause for concern, as this means the individual is at risk of developing diabetes.

Another useful test is the OGTT.

Oral glucose tolerance test

This test measures the body's capacity to utilise glucose and we use this test to make a diagnosis of pre-diabetes, diabetes and gestational diabetes. Prior to the test, the patient eats normally for several days. The patient should not eat or drink anything 8 hours before or during the test. During the OGTT, we measure fasting blood glucose first (see section on fasting blood sugar, above) to establish a baseline level. Second, we ask the patient to drink a liquid which contains about 75 grams of glucose and then take samples of blood every 30–60 minutes. We can take samples for up to 3 hours after ingestion of glucose. During this process, you should reassure your patient but also explain the risk of drawing blood from some people. Such risks include infection, excessive bleeding and blood accumulating under the skin (haematoma). Special consideration should be given to those who are paranoid or confused.

Glucose reading	Condition
Below 8 mmol/L	Normal
8–11 mmol/L	Pre-diabetes
11 mmol/L or higher	Diabetes

Table 5.1: Signifiers for oral glucose tolerance test after 2 hours

For those who do not have type 2 diabetes mellitus or gestational diabetes, the fasting blood glucose values for a 75-gram OGTT should be 3–6 mmol/L initially, then less than 11 mmol/L after an hour and less than 8 mmol/L after 2 hours. If the blood glucose is higher than normal, this may indicate that the individual has pre-diabetes or diabetes (Table 5.1).

Factors that influence the results of an OGTT include second-generation antipsychotics such as olanzapine, risperidone and quetiapine. These drugs may induce glucose intolerance. Before you read further, please take part in this activity.

Activity 5.4   *Evidence-based practice and research*

Alone or in a group, find out which other medicines can induce glucose intolerance in people.

Primary and secondary prevention of type 2 diabetes mellitus

As we have discussed in Chapter 4, the best approach to any disease is to prevent people from having it in the first place. In this regard, it is best to carry out primary prevention. We define primary prevention as prevention of modifiable risk factors by manipulating the social and environmental conditions in which these factors develop. You should discuss with all patients at risk the benefit of a healthy lifestyle that includes healthy diet and exercise and lifestyle changes (see Chapter 3).

Treatment of acute diabetes

Case study

Priya is a 54-year-old woman of South-East Asian origin. She has suffered from depression and anxiety for the past 16 years. Four years after her diagnosis, she developed type 2 diabetes mellitus.

> *Her medication is venlafaxine, gliclazide MR and metformin 500 mg daily. Three days ago she was taken to accident and emergency (A&E) after being found unconscious (Glasgow scale 7) in her house by a neighbour. At A&E, her blood glucose was 1.7 mmol/L. Priya was given a bolus injection of 50 mL with 35% glucose followed by an intravenous infusion of 10% glucose solution. She recovered fully half an hour after correction of hypoglycaemia. An hour later, laboratory results confirmed the diagnosis of hypoglycaemia.*

Hypoglycaemia is a condition where the blood glucose level is too low (below 4.0 mmol/L) and it is a medical emergency, as in Priya's case. It is an important complication of diabetes. Evidence suggests that there is a sixfold increase in deaths due to severe hypoglycaemia in comparison to those not experiencing severe hypoglycaemia (Kalra *et al.* 2013).

There are many reasons why individuals with diabetes experience hypoglycaemia. In Priya's case, it is likely that her use of antidepressants such as venlafaxine interferes with glucose metabolism. Other causes of hypoglycaemia are: delaying or missing administering insulin; delaying or missing meals; unplanned physical activity; and drinking large quantities of alcohol or alcohol without food. In some cases, the cause is not obvious (**www.diabetes.co.uk**). Hypoglycaemia can produce many symptoms, and we can divide these into those resulting from an inadequate supply of glucose to the brain (neuroglycopenic), and those resulting from the body's hormonal response to glucose deficiency. These symptoms are summarised in Table 5.2.

Neuroglycopenic	Hormonal response
Difficulty speaking, slurred speech	Sweating
Poor motor coordination, sometimes	Feeling of numbness
mistaken for drunkenness	Hunger
Movement deficit	Nausea, vomiting, abdominal discomfort
Headaches	Headache
Impaired judgement	Shakiness, anxiety, nervousness
Affective (mood) changes	Palpitations and tachycardia
Irritability, combativeness or rage	Pallor, coldness, clamminess
Stupor, coma, abnormal breathing	Dilated pupils (mydriasis)
Seizures	
Memory loss	
Personality change	
Fatigue, weakness, apathy or sleep	
Confusion, light-headedness or dizziness	
Blurred or double vision	
Flashes of light in the field of vision	
Performing acts without conscious thought	
or intention (automatism)	

Table 5.2: Symptoms of hypoglycaemia (low blood glucose)

When a person with type 2 diabetes mellitus experiences frequent hunger without other symptoms, this indicates that the blood glucose level is too low. This can happen when the person takes excessive oral hypoglycaemic medication such as metformin, glibenclamide, miglitol or insulin relative to the amount of food s/he eats. The drop in blood glucose level to below the normal range triggers a hunger response, although this response is not as marked as in type 1 diabetes.

Bear in mind that not all of the symptoms in Table 5.2 would occur in every individual with hypoglycaemia. However, if you notice some of the symptoms in someone with diabetes, you should treat this as an emergency. The first thing to do is to confirm the diagnosis by testing the blood sugar level using a glucometer. If the patient is confused, you should let the Mental Capacity Act 2005 guide you. If the blood glucose level is low, then treatment usually involves raising the blood glucose level to normal as soon as possible. The patient can achieve this in minutes by taking 10–20 grams of carbohydrates (**www.diabetes.co.uk**). Encourage the patient to take glucose (e.g. about 120 mL of orange or apple juice, four teaspoonfuls of sugar or one slice of bread), whichever is to hand and whatever the patient is able to swallow. Avoid giving the patient chocolate, as it does not work quickly enough due to its high fat content.

The patient's symptoms normally start to improve within 5 minutes and a full recovery may take up to 20 minutes. You should check the blood glucose level 15 minutes later. If it is still below normal, give the patient a further glucose source and wait another 15 minutes before checking blood glucose levels. Meanwhile, you can check the patient's vital signs and observe for conscious-ness, alertness and orientation. Always reassure your patient and explain what you are doing. If the patient has not responded after a second dose of glucose, you should call for an ambulance.

If the hypoglycaemic episode is such that the patient is now unable to take anything orally, as happened to Priya, then we need to give the patient an intramuscular injection of glucagon. As we discussed earlier, glucagon is a hormone that causes a rapid conversion of glycogen to glucose in the liver. The individual should start to respond within minutes and the response can last up to 90 minutes. Whilst your patient is responding to the effects of glucagon, and the blood glucose levels are within a safe range, you should encourage the patient to eat a more sustainable source of glucose (e.g. slices of bread or fruit juice). If glucagon is not available and the patient is not able to take anything by mouth, contact the ambulance services (by dialling 999) immediately after putting the patient in a recovery position. Establish an intravenous route for glucose admin-istration as soon as possible.

Going back to Priya's case, because of her physical condition, the treatment of choice would be an injection of 50 mL with 35% glucose, followed by an intravenous infusion of 10% glucose solution.

Another complication of diabetes is the opposite of hypoglycaemia, the condition we call hyperglycaemia.

Hyperglycaemia

Case study

Chris is a 67-year-old male from Wales and he has suffered from schizophrenia since he was 27 years old; he has been taking risperidone for the past 10 years. Five years ago, he was diagnosed with type 2 diabetes mellitus and takes glicazide and metformin. Three days ago, he was found wandering in the street late at night and appeared confused, complaining of thirst, frequent urination, headaches, lethargy and abdominal pains. He was taken to hospital, where his blood glucose level was 21 mmol/L, with high ketones. Ketones are substances that are made when the body breaks down fat for energy. Glycated haemoglobin (HbA1c) was checked and was 8.5%. Chris's condition was immediately treated with insulin injection and he was also prescribed an oral hypoglycaemic medicine, pramlintide.

A key characteristic of hyperglycaemia is excessively high glucose levels of 11 mmol/L or above. In Chris's case, his blood glucose levels are 21 mmol/L, which shows that he is hyperglycaemic. The cause of hyperglycaemia is usually due to low insulin levels and/or resistance to insulin, depending on the type and state of the disease. Low levels of insulin or resistance to insulin prevent the conversion of glucose into glycogen and this failure leads to glucose accumulating in the blood to abnormally high levels. Several situations increase the risk of hyperglycaemia and these include:

- certain drugs, like beta-blockers, diuretics, noradrenaline, thiazide, corticosteroids, niacin, pentamidine, protease inhibitors, L-asparaginase and second-generation antipsychotic agents, as is likely in Chris's case;

- patients suffering from stroke, acute stress or myocardial infarction, even in the absence of a formal diagnosis of diabetes;

- infection and inflammation can cause hyperglycaemia. When the body is under stress, it releases endogenous catecholamines which raise the blood glucose level in the body.

Signs and symptoms of hyperglycaemia

In most cases, temporary hyperglycaemia causes relatively little harm and the sufferer shows no symptoms. However, chronic hyperglycaemia over a number of years can produce a wide range of serious complications that include kidney, neurological, cardiovascular and retinal damage as well as damage to the feet and legs. Additionally, diabetic neuropathy may be a long term complication of hyperglycaemia. In this regard, it is important to recognise the symptoms of hyperglycaemia (Table 5.3).

Excessive thirst (polydipsia)

Excessive urination (polyuria)

Excessive hunger or increased appetite (polyphagia)

Blurred vision

Fatigue

Dry mouth

Weight loss

Poor wound healing

Dry or itchy skin

Tingling in feet or heels

Erectile dysfunction

Recurrent infections

Cardiac arrhythmia

Stupor

Coma

Seizures

Table 5.3: Symptoms of hyperglycaemia (raised blood glucose)

Before you read further, please take part in the next activity.

Activity 5.5   *Critical thinking*

Chris is a 28-year-old man who suffers from schizophrenia and asthma. He has recently been treated with noradrenaline after an asthmatic attack. What would be your concern about Chris's treatment?

If hyperglycaemia is due to lack of insulin, this can lead to a condition we call diabetic ketoacidosis (DKA), a serious condition that can lead to a diabetic coma or death in extreme cases. DKA is common in those with type 1 diabetes mellitus but it can also be seen in those with type 2 diabetes. If the hyperglycaemia leads to DKA, the body cells are not getting energy from glucose because there is insufficient insulin to facilitate glucose entry into the cells. The body cells will then resort to metabolising fat (lipids) to get energy. Unfortunately, one of the byproducts of fat metabolism is ketones. Ketones are acidic and when they build up in the body, they become toxic to the body cells, which then fail to function properly. For this reason, always check for the presence of ketones in your patient's urine when the blood glucose level is above 12 mmol/L or when the patient has an infection. During periods of infection, the body responds by producing more glucose.

Advise the patient not to exercise, as this will only metabolise more fat, causing more ketones in the body. This can be a particular problem in patients who are agitated because of psychosis or depression. Normally, DKA develops slowly but, when vomiting occurs, this usually means the patient is likely to experience a DKA attack in a few hours and therefore you should contact the doctor if some of the symptoms below accompany the vomiting:

- altered mental status; this may be difficult to detect in patients who are confused or agitated;
- neurological signs, including focal signs such as sensory or motor impairment or focal seizures or motor abnormalities, including flaccidity, depressed reflexes, tremors or **fasciculations**. These symptoms can be confused with signs and symptoms of lithium toxicity;
- **hyperviscosity syndrome** and increased risk of thrombosis;
- polydipsia.

As previously mentioned, DKA is a medical emergency and, if there is no prompt treatment, it can lead to death. The treatment of DKA usually involves giving the patient oral or intravenous fluids to replace fluid lost due to excessive urination. Intravenous rehydration is a critical part of treating DKA because not only does it replace extravascular and intravascular fluids, it also replenishes electrolyte losses. Further, rehydration helps to dilute the glucose in the blood. To correct the fluid lost, we tend to use either isotonic sodium chloride solution or **Lactated Ringer's solution**. When blood glucose decreases to less than 10 mmol/L, we can replace isotonic sodium chloride solution with 5–10% dextrose with half isotonic sodium chloride solution. We can then initiate insulin therapy about an hour after intravenous fluid replacement. Please note that there is little or no advantage in starting insulin therapy before rehydration and evaluation of serum potassium levels (see below). We only use low-dose short-acting insulin for the treatment of DKA to avoid inducing hypoglycaemia or **hypokalaemia** that we see in high-dose insulin treatment. The intravenous or intramuscular route is preferable to the subcutaneous route in people with DKA, as dehydration reduces subcutaneous absorption of insulin.

A second complication of diabetes mellitus, especially type 2 diabetes mellitus, is the hyperosmolar hyperglycaemic state (HHS). In this condition, pancreatic insulin is not effective in controlling blood glucose and therefore blood glucose levels rise. To correct this imbalance, the body then tries to get rid of the excess glucose by excreting it through the urine. This requires excessive urination, which leads to severe dehydration. In turn, severe dehydration can cause complications such as coma or death. Because insulin is present in HHS, there are no ketones found in the urine. In contrast to DKA, the blood glucose level in HHS is extremely high (greater than 33 mmol/L), but ketones are absent or present mildly (Table 5.4). The individual is more likely to experience an alteration in mental status in HHS than DKA. It is a serious condition and is common in older people. Therefore, it is good practice to check for blood glucose levels in older people when they appear confused and restless. Such patients are unlikely to communicate their symptoms effectively to the nurse. For this reason, you have to rely mostly on your observational skills. Before you read further, please take part in the next activity.

Activity 5.6   *Critical thinking*

Percy is a 27-year-old man who suffers from schizoaffective disorder and recently, his medication was switched to haloperidol depot injection after a diagnosis of type 2 diabetes. Two days ago, he had his depot injection just before lunch. About an hour later, the nursing staff noticed that he was confused and restless and his temperature was 39°C. What two conditions could Percy be suffering from and how would you distinguish between the two?

Blood sugar level over 33.3 mmol/L

Dry, parched mouth

Extreme thirst (although this may gradually disappear)

Warm, dry skin that does not sweat

High fever (over 38.3°C)

Sleepiness or confusion

Loss of vision

Hallucinations

Weakness on one side of the body

Table 5.4: Signs and symptoms of hyperosmolar hyperglycaemic state

Essentially, the treatment of HHS consists of rehydrating the patient with intravenous fluids and reducing the blood glucose levels with insulin. This care should include airway management and care of the unconscious. If you are considering inserting an intravenous catheter for rehydration, you should use one with a large bore if possible. In particular, you should consider inserting a central venous line as it offers an avenue for vigorous rehydration.

Fluid deficiency in people with HHS is substantial and may be 10 litres or more in adults. If a recent record of the patient's weight is available for comparison, the difference between the admission weight and the preadmission weight may provide a rough estimate of the degree of dehydration. The treatment goal is to infuse enough fluids so that there is sufficient perfusion in vital organs such as the liver, kidney and brain. In this regard, it is reasonable to replace half of the volume deficit estimate in the first 12 hours of treatment. You can then replace the remainder of the volume deficit over the second 12-hour period. For all adults with clinical dehydration, we consider 0.9% isotonic saline to be appropriate, though some clinicians recommend changing to half-normal saline after a time.

All patients with HHS require intravenous insulin therapy, but immediate treatment with insulin is inadvisable in the initial management. This is because glucose exerts an osmotic pressure within the vascular space which contributes to circulation maintenance in the severely dehydrated patient. If you start insulin therapy without first replacing fluids, this will drive glucose, potassium and water into cells, causing circulatory collapse.

Once the kidneys show evidence of perfusion (urine output), it is safe to initiate insulin therapy. Infuse insulin separately from other fluids and, once you start insulin therapy, do not interrupt or suspend the infusion.

All patients who have experienced HHS will probably require intensive management of their diabetes initially, and this includes insulin therapy. The severe hyperglycaemia with which these patients present implies profound beta-cell dysfunction. In most instances, sufficient recovery of endogenous insulin production is a reasonable expectation, with safe discharge of the patient from the hospital on oral therapy. After maintaining adequate glycaemic control with insulin for several weeks after HHS, it is reasonable to switch the patient to an oral regimen.

Oral glucose control agents

There are at least six distinct classes of hypoglycaemic medicines currently available and each class shows unique pharmacological properties. These classes are the sulphonylureas, meglitinides, biguanides, thiazolidinediones and alpha-glucosidase inhibitors, and we will go on to discuss each of these. When a patient with type 2 diabetes mellitus does not respond to diet and exercise in controlling the condition, we may wish to try one oral medication. Because of the apparently progressive nature of the beta-cell defect in type 2 diabetes, current oral therapies may not prevent an eventual decline in glycaemic control, and it is likely that many patients will ultimately require insulin therapy. Once we make the decision to initiate therapy with an oral medicine, it is wise to consider some patient-specific factors such as age, weight, level of glycaemic control and medicine-specific characteristics (relative potencies, duration of action, side-effect profiles, cost) to make the most appropriate choice (Luna and Feinglos 2001).

The first group of antidiabetic medicines to discuss are sulphonylureas.

Sulphonylureas

This is a class of antidiabetic medicines that we use in the management of type 2 diabetes mellitus. They work by increasing insulin release from the beta cells of the pancreas and may lessen insulin resistance. They have been the main antidiabetic therapy for the past 50 years or so. Older-generation sulphonylureas such as tolazamide and chlorpropamide are just as effective as the newer generation, such as glipizide and glimepiride. However, the newer-generation sulphonylureas have a more favourable side-effect profile. In this respect, we should base our prescribing decision on patient tolerability of the medicine. In a patient who is not responding at one-half the maximum dose, we should consider an alternative agent or combination therapy such as meglitinides.

Meglitinides

Meglitinides work similarly to sulphonylureas and reduce blood sugar levels by increasing insulin production by the pancreas. Unlike the sulphonylureas, they have a very short onset of action (15–30 minutes) and short half-life and therefore must be taken several times a day. Common meglitinides are repaglinide and nateglinide. One potential advantage of this class of medicine is their minimal risk of inducing hypoglycaemia.

Another option for the oral treatment of diabetes is biguanides.

Biguanides

These lower blood sugar in two ways. First, they reduce the conversion of glycogen to glucose by the liver. Second, they increase the amount of glucose the muscle cells absorb and enhance insulin sensitivity. In addition, they can decrease levels of low-density lipoprotein cholesterol (LDL-C: bad cholesterol) and triglycerides more than other diabetes medications.

Metformin is currently the main medicine in this class and reduces HbA1c levels by approximately 1.5–2.0%. One advantage of metformin is that it does not induce hypoglycaemia if used as monotherapy. However, in combination with sulphonylureas or insulin, it can induce hypoglycaemia. Metformin is unique among the oral antidiabetic medicines in that it does not cause weight gain and it can even cause weight loss in some patients. This makes it an ideal oral antidiabetic for those with weight problems, especially those on second-generation antipsychotics.

A fourth class of oral antidiabetic medication is thiazolidinediones.

Thiazolidinediones

These medicines work by promoting insulin sensitivity in the muscle and fat tissues, especially when we use them with other antidiabetic drugs. To a lesser extent, they inhibit the liver from producing glucose. Monotherapy use of thiazolidiniones can reduce HbA1c levels by up to 1.5% and alter lipid profiles by reducing LDL and triglycride levels by as much as 33%.

The last group of antidiabetic medication to discuss is the alpha-glucosidase inhibitors.

Alpha-glucosidase inhibitors

Alpha-glucosidase inhibitors work by stopping the action of the enzyme alpha-glucosidase. This enzyme normally catalyses the breakdown of complex carbohydrates to glucose in the small intestine. They can reduce HbA1c by up to 1.0%. Acarbose and miglitol are the two medicines available in this class.

General care and tertiary prevention

Case study

Jane is a 45-year-old woman who lives with her husband and two teenage children. She suffers from bipolar disorder and, about 9 months ago, she was diagnosed with type 2 diabetes. At presentation, she was experiencing polyuria, blurry vision and a random glucose level of 15 mmol/L. Her HbA1c at that time was 8.0%. She was prescribed metformin 500 mg twice daily, and within 3 months, her HbA1c dropped to 7.6%. The metformin was increased further to 1000 mg twice daily. She had been partially adherent with her treatment as she often forgets to take her medication on time. She reports that her home blood sugar readings have improved slightly but are still high. She admits to a few dietary indiscretions, such as having multiple servings of dessert when going out with friends. She acknowledges the value of engaging in regular exercise but has not been active.

Tertiary prevention is a level of preventive care that deals with the rehabilitation and return of a patient to a status of maximum usefulness with a minimum risk of recurrence of the disorder. By extension, this involves a degree of self-care. The National Institute for Health and Care Excellence (NICE) guideline recommends that the management of people with diabetes should involve a degree of self-care (NICE 2009b). We should therefore configure our approach to fit in with the needs and preferences of our patients suffering from diabetes. Where possible and with the consent of the patient, we should involve their carers. In Jane's example, it is important to involve her husband and children in the overall care.

In partnership with the patient, you should give the opportunity for the patient to make informed decisions about care and treatment. However, if you suspect that the person may not have the capacity to make decisions, then the Mental Capacity Act 2005 should guide you in your decision making. It is essential that you establish good communication between the patient and yourself. You should always ensure that the information you give the patient fits the patient's educational level and is culturally sensitive. The information you give must be accessible to mental health patients with physical, sensory or learning disabilities, and to people who do not speak or read English. At times, you may need to offer the information repeatedly to patients as many patients with psychosis, depression and Alzheimer's disease may have cognitive deficits that interfere with assimilating information. According to NICE (2009b) guidelines, these are the key areas of intervention in tertiary prevention:

- You should offer structured education to every person and/or carer at and around the time of diagnosis, with annual reinforcement and review. Inform people and their carers that structured education is a necessary part of diabetes care.

- You should provide personalised and ongoing nutritional advice, preferably from a dietician. Please refer to Chapter 9.

- You should involve the individual in setting an HbA1c target level, which may be above that of 6.5% set for people with type 2 diabetes in general:

  - Encourage people to maintain their individual target unless the resulting side effects (including hypoglycaemia) or their efforts to achieve this impair their quality of life.

  - Offer therapy (lifestyle and medication) to help achieve and maintain the HbA1c target level.

  - Inform a person with a higher HbA1c that any reduction in HbA1c towards the agreed target is advantageous to future health.

  - Avoid pursuing highly intensive management to levels of less than 6.5%.

- You should discuss the purpose of self-monitoring of plasma glucose to a person with a recent diagnosis of type 2 diabetes. This should be integral to the patient's self-management education.

- When a patient is starting insulin therapy, you should use a structured programme employing active insulin dose titration that encompasses:

  - structured education;

  - continuing telephone support;

  - frequent self-monitoring;

  - dose titration to target;

  - dietary understanding;

  - management of hypoglycaemia;

  - management of acute changes in plasma glucose control;

  - support from an appropriately trained and experienced healthcare professional.

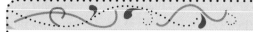

Chapter summary

Metabolic syndrome is a collection of several risk factors for cardiovascular disease and diabetes. It is characterised by any three of the following: increase in abdominal fat, high blood triglycerides, high levels of LDL, low HDL, high blood pressure and high fasting blood glucose. Metabolic syndrome is very common in people with mental health problems, in comparison to the general population. By extension, the prevalence of type 2 diabetes is disproportionately high in people with mental health problems. We attribute much of this risk to a variety of factors, including genetic and lifestyle but, most importantly of all, the use of psychotropic medication.

Successful management of diabetes usually includes a combination of pharmacological and lifestyle change interventions. With regard to pharmacological interventions, the common medicines in use are sulphonylureas, meglitinides, biguanides, thiazolidinediones and alpha-glucosidase inhibitors. Non-pharmacological interventions such as dietary advice and exercise often accompany pharmacological interventions. In the treatment of diabetes, the empowerment of the patient and carers is critical to the successful resolution of the condition.

Activities: brief outline answers

Activity 5.1

The blood glucose level is likely to be high (above normal) and therefore unlikely to reflect the normal blood glucose level for that patient.

Activity 5.2

Aripiprazole, asenapine, iloperidone, fluoxetine and citalopram.

Activity 5.3

Blurred vison (side effect of antipsychotics and antidepressants), feeling tired, increased thirst (depression or negative symptoms of schizophrenia) and tingling sensations (schizophrenia).

Activity 5.4

Beta-blockers (for example, propranolol), birth control pills, corticosteroids (for example, prednisone), dextrose, noradrenaline, oestrogens, glucagon, isoniazid, lithium, phenothiazines, phenytoin, salicylates (including aspirin), thiazide diuretics (for example, hydrochlorothiazide), triamterene, tricyclic antidepressants. In addition to drugs, acute stress and vigorous exercise can alter the results of an OGTT.

Activity 5.5

Chris is at risk of developing stress hyperglycaemia because noradrenaline tends to elevate glucose levels in the blood, causing stress hyperglycaemia.

Activity 5.6

Some symptoms of HHS overlap with those of neuroleptic malignancy syndrome (NMS). These symptoms include high temperature and confusion, tachycardia and hallucinations. If blood glucose is more than 33 mmol/L, then the condition is likely to be HHS. If high temperature accompanies labile blood pressure, then the condition is likely to be NMS.

Further reading

Challem J, Burton B, Smith MD (2000) *Syndrome X.* Chichester: John Wiley.

A detailed book that explains metabolic syndrome and its complications in accessible style.

Collins E, Drake M, Deacon M (2013) *Physical Care of People with Mental Health Problems.* London: Sage.

This book covers key areas of interest, particularly for people with mental health problems.

Nash M (2010) *Physical Health and Well Being in Mental Health Nursing: Clinical skills for practice.* Maidenhead, Berkshire: McGraw-Hill Open University.

A concise book that covers the main areas of physical health in people with mental health problems.

Cormac I, Gray D (2012) *Essentials of Physical Health in Psychiatry.* London: RCPsych publications.

A more detailed book on the treatment of physical health problems for people with mental health problems. Suitable for those with an interest in the diagnosis and treatment of diseases.

Useful websites

http://www.nhs.uk/Conditions/Diabetes

Useful, complete with case histories and expert opinions and suitable for carers, sufferers and professionals.

http://www.diabetes.org.uk

Useful information, particularly for service users and their families. Has instructions on what do to in different scenarios.

http://www.diabetes.org

Website for the American Diabetes Association; has very useful information.

Chapter 6
Respiratory disorders

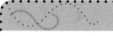
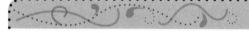
Chapter aims

By the end of the chapter, you should be able to:

- understand and describe chronic obstructive pulmonary disorder;
- discuss the risk factors associated with respiratory disorders;
- discuss primary, secondary and tertiary interventions for respiratory disorder.

Introduction

Case study

Raheem is a 59-year-old male with a 30-year history of depression and he smokes 30 cigarettes a day. Over the past 5 years, he has become increasingly short of breath. Initially, he noticed this only when he was exercising, but recently he runs out of breath even if he is at rest. Raheem has had several bouts of lower respiratory tract infection which have been treated successfully with antibiotics over the past 2 years. His experience of shortness of breath has not subsided and his breathing is assisted by the use of his accessory muscles of respiration.

Respiratory disease describes pathological conditions affecting the organs and tissues that make gaseous exchange possible in people. As in the case of Raheem above, the disease affects the upper respiratory tract, consisting of mouth, nose, pharynx and larynx; the second part that this condition affects is the lower respiratory tract, consisting of lungs, trachea, bronchi, bronchioles, alveoli, pleura and pleural cavity (Figure 6.1).

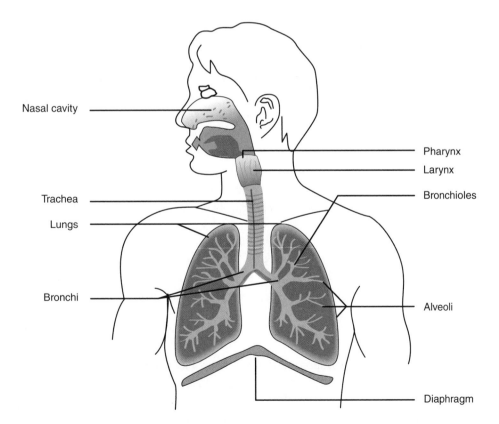

Figure 6.1: Parts of the pulmonary system affected in lung disease

There are several broad categories of respiratory disease: asthma, chronic obstructive pulmonary disease (COPD), pneumonia, tuberculosis and lung cancer. This chapter will discuss the common respiratory diseases of asthma, COPD and pneumonia. We will start with asthma.

Asthma

Asthma is a chronic lung disease that narrows and inflames the airways. It causes recurring periods of a whistling sound when a person breathes, chest tightness, shortness of breath and coughing. More often than not, the coughing occurs at night or early in the morning. According to the World Health Organization (WHO), asthma is a major non-communicable disease and its symptoms can vary in severity and frequency from person to person (WHO 2003a). It is the most common long-term medical condition, affecting approximately 300 million people worldwide, and its prevalence is steadily increasing, especially in westernised societies. In the UK, there are 5.4 million people receiving treatment for asthma, approximately 1.1 million of whom are children (Amlani *et al.* 2011). According to the UK's Department of Health there are around 1,000 deaths a year from asthma and 40% of these are under the age of 75 years. Approximately 90% of these deaths are preventable. Asthma is responsible for large numbers of hospital admissions and about 70% of them are emergencies that are preventable with appropriate early interventions (Department of Health 2011). Many of the emergency admissions are of people with mental health problems.

Asthma and mental health

The association between asthma and psychological factors has been present for centuries and, for a long time, asthma was classified as a psychosomatic disease. In the 1930s–1950s, it was known as one of the 'holy seven' psychosomatic illnesses. At the time, psychoanalytic theories described the aetiology of asthma as psychological, with treatment often primarily involving psychoanalysis and other talking therapies. The asthmatic wheeze was interpreted as the child's suppressed cry for the mother and treatment of depression was viewed as especially important for individuals with asthma. Nowadays, we consider asthma to be a respiratory condition that affects the airways and people with mental health problems are more likely to suffer from asthma than the general population.

One of the earliest empirical findings linking mental health disorders and asthma was by Wamboldt *et al.* (1996). The investigators noted a disproportionately high number of mental health problems, including depression, anxiety and personality disorder, in relatives of children with asthma, therefore indirectly supporting a familial link between severe asthma and various mental health disorders.

Prevalence of depression and asthma comorbidity is up to 45% (Mancuso *et al.* 2001) and further evidence suggests that individuals with asthma are more likely to be depressed than those without (Kovacs *et al.* 2003). Moreover, more severe asthma is directly proportional to more severe depressive symptoms (Mrazek 1992). In addition to depression and anxiety, there is a strong link between asthma and schizophrenia (Schoepf *et al.* 2014). Before we discuss this, please take part in the activity below.

Activity 6.1   *Evidence-based practice and research*

Alone or in a group, find out about any allergic conditions that have an association with mental illness.

There are outline answers to all the activities at the end of the chapter.

There is a growing body of evidence suggesting that asthma significantly increases the risk for schizophrenia (Chen *et al.* 2009; Weber *et al.* 2009; Pedersen *et al.* 2012). Furthermore, a recent prospective longitudinal study that examined this relationship found that the presence of atopic disorders such as asthma increases the risk of psychotic experiences in adolescence (Khandaker *et al.* 2014). Thus, asthma and schizophrenia might share a pathophysiological process, most likely through the immune process. A possible explanatory mechanism is that the excess immune response seen in asthma is also present in schizophrenia. The inflammation which usually accompanies excess immune response may increase the permeability of the blood–brain barrier. This makes the brain vulnerable to immune components like **cytokines** and antibodies, therefore contributing to the development of schizophrenia (Watanabe *et al.* 2010). Clearly, the link between asthma and some mental health problems is evident and we need to understand the causes of asthma.

Risk factors for asthma

Currently, it is not clear what causes asthma, but the hygiene hypothesis formulated by Strachan (1989) may partly explain the aetiology of the condition. The theory suggests that a lack of early childhood exposure to pathogens suppresses the natural development of the immune system and this results in an increase in the susceptibility to allergic diseases. Specifically, the lack of exposure leads to defects in establishing a tolerant immune system. Our western lifestyle emphasises hygiene and sanitation and this has resulted in reduced exposure to pathogens in early childhood (Strachan 2000). Many young children no longer have the same type of environmental exposures to infections as children in the past. This affects the way that young children's immune systems develop during very early childhood, and it may increase their risk for atopy and asthma. The risk factors for asthma are:

- an inherited tendency to develop allergies (atopy);
- having parents with asthma;
- having certain respiratory infections during childhood;
- contact with some airborne allergens or exposure to some viral infections in early childhood during immune system development.

Asthma triggers

The symptoms of asthma can have a range of triggers, but they do not affect everyone in the same way. What is clearer is that genetic and environmental factors interact to trigger asthma, most often early in life. These may include any of the following ten types of trigger.

Airway and chest infections

Flu and viruses often cause upper respiratory infections, which trigger asthma. Airway and chest infections are common in people with mental health problems; therefore, it is not surprising that this should trigger asthma in this population (see later sections).

Allergens

Pollen, dust mites, animal fur or feathers, for example, can trigger asthma. These allergens are common in poor housing conditions. Because of a lack of employment opportunities, people with mental health problems are more likely to live in poor housing conditions, thus increasing the chances of triggering asthma.

Airborne irritants

There is extensive evidence suggesting that cigarette smoking plays a key role in the onset of both childhood and adult asthma. As such, exposure to prenatal smoking appears to be a potential risk factor for asthma and mental health disorders (Weissman *et al.* 1999). Smoking is very common in people with mental health problems, making it more likely to trigger asthma (see Chapter 7). Other airborne irritants that trigger asthma are chemical fumes and atmospheric pollutions.

Medicines

Approximately 10–20% of adults in the general population with asthma are sensitive to aspirin or to painkillers we call non-steroidal anti-inflammatory drugs (NSAIDs). These medicines include ibuprofen, naproxen and aspirin. Asthma attacks due to any of these medications can be severe or even fatal. It is therefore important that patients should completely avoid these medicines if they have a known aspirin-sensitive asthma. To a lesser extent, beta-blockers and angiotensin-converting enzyme inhibitors (see Chapter 4) trigger asthma and a significant number of people with mental health problems are likely to be taking these medicines.

Emotional factors

Emotional factors such as stress can trigger asthma. There is extensive evidence suggesting that family functioning plays a key role in asthma and adolescents living in high expressed emotion households respond better to treatment when separated from their parents. Incidentally, people living in high expressed emotion households tend to experience poorer mental health recovery.

Sulphite-containing foods

Sulphites are naturally occurring substances in food and drinks that we use as food preservatives. Food and drinks that are rich in sulphites include concentrated fruit juice, jam, prawns and many processed or pre-cooked meals. Sulphites trigger attacks in a significant proportion of people with asthma; also, certain wines can trigger asthma in susceptible people. It is therefore important to inform asthmatic patients of the risks that food preservatives present.

Weather conditions

A sudden change in temperature, cold air, windy days, poor air quality and hot, humid days are all known triggers for asthma.

Indoor conditions

House dust, mites, pets, fungi, insects, mould or damp and chemicals in carpets and flooring materials may trigger asthma. These indoor factors are of particular interest because globally, people spend more than 80% of their time indoors (Heinrich 2011). People with mental health conditions, including depression and schizophrenia, spend even greater amounts of time indoors than the general population. This puts them at an even greater risk of an asthmatic attack than the general population.

Exercise

Among persons with asthma, exercise-induced wheeze is a common symptom. Approximately 40–77% of people with asthma show exercise-induced **bronchoconstriction** (Leichsenring *et al.* 2009). They find that their symptoms worsen when they exercise. Some of the symptoms they show are non-asthmatic inspiratory wheeze, vocal cord dysfunction and **cardiac arrhythmias**, which could limit their physical capacity.

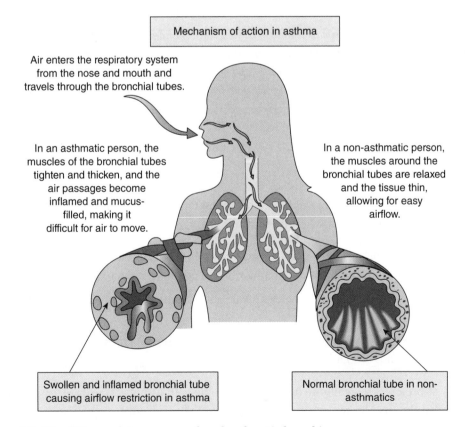

Figure 6.2: The difference between normal and asthmatic bronchi

Food allergies

Although uncommon, some people may have allergies to nuts or other food items, known as an anaphylactic reaction. If so, these can trigger severe asthma attacks.

Asthma mechanism

To understand asthma, we need to understand how the airways work. The relevant airways are tubes of the lower respiratory tract which consist of trachea, bronchi, bronchioles, lungs, alveoli, pleura and pleural cavity. They help to carry air into and out of the lungs. In people with asthma, there is inflammation in these airways, making them swollen and very sensitive. The airways tend to react adversely to certain substances we breathe in. When they react, the muscles around the airways tighten and they become narrower (Figure 6.2). This narrowing causes less air to flow into the lungs. The swelling of the airways can also worsen, making them even narrower. The cells lining the airways may produce excessive mucus that can narrow the airways further.

This sequence of events can result in symptoms of asthma and we will turn to these now.

Signs and symptoms of acute asthma

Case study

Mary is a 37-year-old black female who suffers from anxiety and asthma. Whilst on the ward during the night, she experienced rapid breathing (tachypnoea), chest tightness and acute shortness of breath with audible wheezing. Additional symptoms included tachycardia, oxygen saturation of 93% and coughing up small amounts of white sputum. The nurse administered salbutamol in a small-volume nebuliser whilst waiting for transfer to a general hospital for further and more detailed investigations.

As we can see from the case study above, one of the commonest signs of asthma is coughing, breathing with a wheeze, shortness of breath and chest tightness. Mary has at least three of these symptoms. Let us look more closely at these symptoms.

- Coughing: asthmatic cough is often worse during the night or early in the morning, as we have seen from Mary, and it can make it hard for the patient to sleep.
- Wheezing is a high-pitched whistling or squeaky sound that occurs when a person with asthma breathes, and Mary has this symptom.
- Chest tightness: this is another common symptom of asthma. Typically, the chest tightness feels like something is squeezing or sitting on the chest.

Shortness of breath is a common complaint of people with asthma, as with Mary. Individuals complain that they feel breathless or cannot get air out of their lungs.

Not all people who have asthma have these symptoms and the best way a doctor may diagnose asthma is to perform a lung function test, take the medical history and perform a physical examination.

The diagnosis of asthma

In the diagnosis of asthma, it is important to assess the severity of the condition – whether it is intermittent, mild, moderate or severe. The treatment of asthma depends on the level of severity. Severe symptoms of asthma can be fatal and the severity depends on the type of symptoms a person is experiencing, and how often they occur. This can change over time; therefore, it is important for you to help your patient when you first notice symptoms to prevent them from becoming severe. In Mary's case, the nurse administered salbutamol as an immediate measure to prevent worsening of the asthma, and we will discuss this in detail in later sections. From a diagnostic perspective, the doctor is likely to ask about the history of asthma, or allergies in the family, when symptoms occur, and how often they occur.

In your interactions with the patient, it is important to find out whether symptoms happen during certain times of the year, in certain places, or if symptoms get worse at night, as in the case of Mary. Find out factors that seem to trigger the patient's symptoms or worsen them, such as specific foods, age and gender. For example, those with asthma that is difficult to control tend to be older women, who have poor lung function, are obese and have anxiety or depression (Di *et al.* 2010). Because Mary suffers from anxiety and she is female, we can expect her asthma to be difficult to control. Other conditions that can make the asthma difficult to control are a runny nose, sinus infections, **gastro-oesophageal reflux disease**, psychological stress and sleep apnoea. One definitive test for asthma is the lung function test, but before we discuss this, please take part in the activity below.

Activity 6.2   *Critical thinking*

Judy is a 20-year-old university student studying biochemistry. She suffers from bipolar disorder and asthma. Recently, she has been revising for an important exam and has noticed that she feels very tired during the day. This is because she is unable to sleep well during the night because she coughs frequently. Why do you think Judy is coughing more at night lately and what other complications might you expect?

Lung function test

A key diagnostic test for asthma that checks lung functioning is spirometry (see Chapter 2). Briefly, the test measures how much air a person breathes in and out. It also measures how fast the individual can expel air. Generally a patient is retested after drug treatment to see if the results improve. If the results are lower than normal but improve after taking medicine and the medical history shows a pattern of asthma symptoms, then the person is likely to have asthma.

More than likely, we require further information to make a definite diagnosis of asthma. There are other tests that may be necessary:

- allergy testing;

- a bronchial challenge or broncho-provocation test; this test measures how sensitive the airways are. The test measures lung functioning during physical activity or after the individual receives increasing doses of cold air or a special chemical like methacholine or histamine to breathe in. Both methacholine and histamine provoke narrowing of the airways but histamine also causes nasal and bronchial mucus secretion. We can then quantify the degree of narrowing of the airways using a spirometry test. People with asthma will react to lower doses of the chemicals;

- a test to determine whether an individual has another condition with symptoms similar to that of asthma like reflux disease, vocal cord dysfunction or sleep apnoea;

- a chest X-ray or an electrocardiogram test to determine the presence of a foreign body in the individual's airways or another disease that might be causing symptoms. Your role in diagnosis is to assist the treating team and, most importantly, explain the procedure and reassure your patient.

Once we confirm the diagnosis of asthma, we need to treat the condition at acute and prophylactic level. We will turn to acute asthma first.

Management of acute severe asthma

Case study

Peter has suffered from asthma since he was 9 years old and at 26 he had a diagnosis of schizophrenia. He is divorced and has infrequent access to his young child and lives alone in a flat with two cats. Four days ago, Peter was admitted to hospital with an acute worsening of asthma symptoms. About 3 days before that, he developed a sore throat and nasal catarrh which worsened the wheeze, chest tightness, cough and yellow sputum discharge. He saw his GP, who prescribed antibiotics, but the coughing and wheezing kept him awake at night. Despite taking beta$_2$-agonist medications via his nebuliser at 10:30 hours, his peak flow was 200 L/min, so the community mental health nurse (CMHN) who had visited him called an ambulance to take Peter to hospital. The CMHN phoned Peter's mother who lived nearby to make arrangements for care of the cats.

Asthma is a long-term disease that has no permanent cure. The goal of asthma treatment is to:

- prevent troublesome symptoms, such as coughing and shortness of breath, as with Peter;

- reduce the need for quick-relief medicines like beta-agonists, which Peter uses;

- assist in good lung functioning;

- allow the patient to maintain normal activity levels during the day and be able to sleep during the night. In Peter's case, he is unable to sleep because of coughing and wheezing;

- prevent asthma attacks that may result in emergency admission or hospital stay.

As a nurse, you should be aware that patients with severe asthma who have adverse psychosocial factors are at risk of death (Sturdy *et al.* 2002; Potoczek *et al.* 2006). Those with mental health problems are likely to have adverse psychosocial factors and are therefore at risk of death from an acute severe asthmatic attack. There is also an elevated risk of the patient dying if there is a delay in getting treatment, particularly starting steroid treatment (see later sections).

Other factors that increase the risk of death are a comorbidity with illness such as congestive cardiac failure, COPD (Department of Health 2011) and smoking. Mortality is highest in the very young and the very old. Furthermore, evidence suggests that males of African or Hispanic origin are more likely to suffer from an acute severe asthmatic attack than any other ethnic group (Moore *et al.* 2009). To assist you in deciding what level of intervention you need for those suffering from an acute severe asthmatic attack, see Table 6.1.

Assessment of severity of asthma

Moderate acute asthma

☐ Increasing symptoms
☐ If the peak expiration flow (PEF) is 50–75% of personal best or predicted
☐ No symptoms of acute severe asthma present

Acute severe asthma

This is present in anyone with:

☐ PEF of 33–50% of personal best or predicted
☐ A respiration rate of more than 25 breaths/min
☐ A pulse rate of 110 beats/min or more
☐ Inability to complete sentences in one breath

Life-threatening

We consider a patient's symptoms to be life-threatening if one or more of the following is present:

☐ A PEF of less than 33% of personal best or predicted best
☐ An oxygen saturation (SpO_2) of less than 92%
☐ An oxygen partial pressure (PaO_2) of less than 8 kPa
☐ A normal carbon dioxide partial pressure ($PaCO_2$) of 4.6–6.0 kPa
☐ Silent chest
☐ Cyanosis
☐ Poor respiratory effort
☐ Arrhythmia
☐ Exhaustion and/or altered conscious level

Near-fatal

Raised *Pa*CO_2 or requiring mechanical
ventilation with raised inflation pressures

Table 6.1: Levels of severity of acute asthmatic attack

Depending on the level of severity, you should consider calling the ambulance if the patient is in the community and if in hospital, you should call the doctor or ambulance straight away. Whilst waiting for the doctor or ambulance to arrive, give supplementary oxygen to the patient with acute severe asthma to maintain an Spo_2 level of 94–98%. Even if you have not been able to measure the Spo_2 level, this should not prevent you from giving oxygen to the patient. Typically, asthmatic patients tend to be on beta$_2$-bronchodilators, the most common of which is salbutamol or terbutaline. You should encourage your patient to take a beta$_2$-agonist, usually via a large spacer device or nebuliser. The nebuliser should be oxygen-driven where it is available. In patients where inhalation of beta$_2$-agonist is unreliable during an acute episode of asthma, the doctor may give intravenous beta$_2$-agonists (bronchodilators). It is also common practice to administer ipratropium bromide in addition to the beta$_2$-agonist for those with acute severe or life-threatening asthma, or those with a poor initial response to beta$_2$-agonist therapy. Ipratropium bromide is an anticholinergic medication that inhibits bronchoconstriction and mucus secretion that is common during an acute asthmatic attack. During an acute asthmatic attack, the use of corticosteroids is an important treatment intervention.

Corticosteroids are medicines that decrease inflammation and swelling of the airways, seen in asthma attacks. Corticosteroids reduce mortality and the patient should have these as early as possible during an acute asthmatic attack. Current asthma guidelines suggest that patients should consider decreasing or stopping corticosteroids when the asthma is stable. However, recent evidence from a systematic review of 172 studies suggests that patients with well-controlled asthma who stop regular use of low-dose inhaled corticosteroids are at an elevated risk of their asthma worsening than those who continue to use corticosteroids (Rank *et al.* 2013). Inhaled corticosteroids that are in common use are beclomethasone, fluticasone and budesonide.

For people whose acute asthma is life-threatening, doctors usually give a single dose of intravenous magnesium sulphate. Magnesium sulphate is a potent bronchodilator that is used after beta$_2$-agonist and anticholinergic medicines have been tried in the severe worsening of asthma (Blitz *et al.* 2005). Emerging evidence also supports the use of ketamine in alleviating acute severe asthmatic symptoms. A systematic review of 24 studies found an improvement in outcome with the use of ketamine in acute severe asthma that is not responsive to conventional treatment (Goyal and Agrawal 2013). If there is a failure to manage acute severe asthma correctly, complications can arise, some of which are:

- aspiration pneumonia;
- **pneumomediastinum**;
- **pneumothorax**;
- **rhabdomyolysis**;
- respiratory failure and arrest;
- cardiac arrest;
- hypoxic-ischaemic brain injury;
- death.

Step-up/down management of chronic asthma

In the management of chronic asthma, the British Thoracic Society (2009) recommends stepped-up/stepped-down care, which comprises five steps.

Step 1: Mild, intermittent asthma

For moderate asthma, you should encourage the patient to use the short-acting beta$_2$-agonist as a short-term measure to relieve mild symptoms of asthma.

Step 2: Regular preventer therapy

We add corticosteroid therapy for patients with a recent worsening of asthma (during the past 2 years), those who wake up during the night due to symptoms or those who have daytime symptoms three times or more per week. Inhaled corticosteroids are the most effective preventer medicines for achieving overall treatment goals. The regular use of bronchodilators alone may have an association with worsening asthma and asthma deaths.

Step 3: Add-on therapy

If there is failure to control the asthma fully, the patient should take long-acting beta$_2$-agonists (LABAs) in addition to inhaled steroids. Because LABAs have a long duration of action (up to 12 hours), they reduce the need for shorter-acting beta$_2$-agonists such as salbutamol. However, they are not suitable for the treatment of acute asthma because of their slower onset of action. LABAs in common use are salmeterol and formoterol. If a patient is responsive to the addition of LABAs, then the patient should continue on this medication and you should continue to monitor effectiveness. In some cases, the patient may experience partial effectiveness after addition of LABAs. In this case, an increase of the inhaled steroid dose up to 800 µg/day of beclometasone propionate or equivalent if necessary. If the asthma control is suboptimal after the increase of inhaled steroid, the next stage (Stephens *et al.* 1980) is to consider a trial of another add-on therapy, such as leukotriene receptor antagonists or modified-release theophylline.

Step 4: Poor control on moderate dose of inhaled steroid plus add-on therapy

If the patient's asthma remains under suboptimal control, another add-on therapy at this stage is leukotriene receptor antagonist. Leukotrienes are fatty compounds produced by the immune system and they cause inflammation in bronchitis and asthma. Leukotriene receptor antagonists, such as montelukast, provide a safe and effective treatment option with ease of administration, as add-on therapy in patients with difficult-to-control asthma (Amlani *et al.* 2011). In addition to leukotriene receptor antagonists, it is normal to treat patients with sustained-release theophylline or beta$_2$-agonist tablet. It is usual in stage 4 to increase the dose of inhaled corticosteroid to 2,000 µg/day.

Step 5: Continuous or frequent use of oral steroids

Where previous steps have failed to control a patient's asthma, the use of regular prednisolone is the treatment of choice. At this point, the patient should be under specialist care. The use of oral steroids risks the patient developing side effects that you should monitor and manage. These side effects are hypertension, diabetes or hyperlipidaemia, osteoporosis, cataracts and **adrenal suppression**. If a patient's asthma has been stable for a long time, it may be prudent to consider stepping down care.

Stepping down

It is important to review care and management of asthma every 3 months and if possible to step down the care. However, it is also important to make consideration for variation in symptoms, severity of asthma, risk of adverse effects and patient preference and use the lowest possible dose of inhaled corticosteroid to control the asthma symptoms. Generally, when reducing inhaled steroids, the dose reduction should be slow, by 25–50% each time.

We now need to turn to an equally important aspect of COPD but before we do that, please take part in the activity below.

Activity 6.3   *Critical thinking*

In Peter's example in the earlier case study, what symptoms of depression may interfere with the management of his asthma?

Chronic obstructive pulmonary disease

COPD or chronic obstructive airway disease is a type of lung disease that obstructs the airways, resulting in chronic poor airflow. This limit in airflow usually worsens over time and has a clear association with an abnormal inflammatory response of the lungs to harmful particles or gases. COPD consists of two groups of lung disease – chronic bronchitis and emphysema – and we will discuss these conditions in more detail in later sections. It is the fourth leading cause of morbidity and mortality worldwide, but the WHO predicts it will become the third leading cause of death by 2030 (WHO 2011b). The prevalence of this disease increases with age, but importantly, its association with smoking is clear and dramatic. Smokers have a strikingly higher prevalence and mortality from COPD and related illness than non-smokers (Mannino and Buist 2007).

Until 50 years ago, respiratory diseases, such as pneumonia and tuberculosis, accounted for the majority of deaths amongst people with mental health problems who lived in institutions. The prevalence of COPD is still significantly higher in people with mental health problems in comparison to the general population (Himelhoch *et al.* 2004). In a study of 200 outpatients, 15% of those with schizophrenia and 25% of those with bipolar disorder had chronic bronchitis, and

16% of people with schizophrenia and 19% of people with bipolar disorder had asthma. These rates were significantly higher than the matched controls from the general population. The same study found that, even after controlling for the confounding effects for smoking, emphysema rates were still higher in people with schizophrenia and bipolar disorder.

In the past two decades, a higher incidence of COPD has been associated with the side effects of phenothiazine antipsychotics (Volkov 2009). To enable us to understand COPD, it is important to understand how the lungs work first.

Understanding the mechanism of COPD

When we breathe in air, it goes down the windpipe into the bronchial tubes or airways. Within the lungs, the bronchial tubes branch into thousands of smaller, thinner tubes called bronchioles. These tubes end in tiny round air sacs or alveoli where small blood vessels (capillaries) run through the walls of the air sacs. Gaseous exchange takes place in these alveoli. In a healthy person with no COPD, the airways and air sacs are elastic and when the individual breathes in, each air sac fills up with air like a small balloon. When an individual breathes out, the air sacs deflate and the air goes out, just like a deflating small balloon. In COPD, less air flows in and out of the airways because of one or more of the following:

- The airways and air sacs lose their elasticity, therefore making it difficult to fill them with air.
- The walls between many of the air sacs are destroyed, forming larger and fewer alveoli (Figure 6.3). This reduces the surface area for gaseous exchange.
- The walls of the airways become thick and inflamed and this slows down gaseous exchange.
- The airways (bronchioles) lose shape and make more mucus than usual, which can clog them. Again, this limits surface area for gaseous exchange as well as slowing down the process.

One component of COPD is bronchitis and we will turn our attention to this now.

Bronchitis

Case study

Martin is a 52-year-old man who suffers from schizoaffective disorder and is currently a mental health unit inpatient. He is widowed, lives alone, and has difficulty managing his daily activities. Four years ago, he was diagnosed with chronic bronchitis and attends the chest clinic regularly. He smokes about 30 cigarettes a day. For the past week, he has experienced increased difficulty in breathing (dyspnoea) and cough and has been unable to care for himself. His personal hygiene appears to have deteriorated. He complained of mild nausea without abdominal pain or vomiting. The nurse took his vital signs and they were as follows: blood pressure 190/115 mmHg, pulse rate 125 beats/min, respiratory rate 30 breaths/min and oral temperature 37°C. The nurse contacted the doctor straight away so that Martin could receive further investigations.

Chronic Obstructive Pulmonary Disease (COPD)

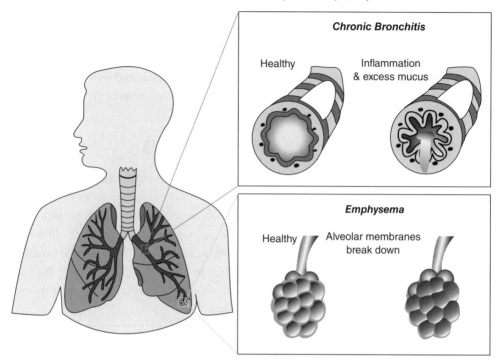

Figure 6.3: The location of the lungs and airways in the body. Inset: detailed cross-section of the bronchioles and alveoli for someone with chronic obstructive pulmonary disease

Bronchitis is an inflammation of the mucous membranes of the bronchi (Figure 6.3). As the irritated mucous membrane swells and grows thicker, it narrows or shuts off the tiny airways in the lungs, resulting in coughing spells that produce phlegm and breathlessness, as in Martin's case study above. The disease comes in two forms: the acute phase, which lasts 1–3 weeks, and the chronic phase, which lasts at least 3 months of the year for 2 years in a row. Martin's bronchitis is in a chronic phase as he has experienced symptoms for 4 years. However, let us discuss acute bronchitis first.

Acute bronchitis

Acute bronchitis is an inflammation of the large airways (trachea, bronchi) of the lung that manifests as cough without pneumonia. The main cause of acute bronchitis is usually viruses from influenza A and B viruses, parainfluenza virus, **respiratory syncytial virus**, **coronavirus**, **adenovirus** and **rhinovirus**. Human **metapneumovirus** has been identified as a causative agent. Quite often, the same viruses that cause colds and flu are the most common cause of acute bronchitis. These viruses spread through the air when people cough and through physical contact such as unwashed hands. In rare circumstances, some bacteria or fungi can cause bronchitis.

As previously mentioned, acute bronchitis lasts from a few days to 10 days but the coughing may last for several weeks after the infection is gone. Several factors increase the risk for acute bronchitis and these include exposure to tobacco smoke (including second-hand smoke), dust, fumes, vapours and air pollution. Therefore, avoiding these lung irritants as much as possible can help lower the risk for acute bronchitis.

Some key symptoms of acute bronchitis are expectorating cough (thick yellow mucus), shortness of breath (dyspnoea) and wheezing. In certain instances, the patient may experience chest pains and fever, and fatigue or malaise may also occur. In addition, bronchitis caused by *Adenoviridae* may cause systemic and gastrointestinal symptoms. However, coughs due to bronchitis can continue for up to 3 weeks or more, even after all other symptoms have subsided.

Because bronchitis is usually due to a viral infection, its treatment with antibiotics is ineffective. A key treatment priority is to lower the temperature and the inflammation and for this, the patient can take ibuprofen or paracetamol. The patient can take cough expectorants to help loosen mucus in the lungs and make it easier to cough up. This can make breathing easier. Additionally, the patient can take cough-suppressant medication if the cough is not producing mucus. Care for acute bronchitis may consist of simple measures such as encouraging the patient to get plenty of rest, drink plenty of fluids and avoid smoke and fumes. As previously discussed, if acute bronchitis lasts for longer than 3 months, it becomes chronic.

Chronic bronchitis

If there is ongoing irritation and inflammation of the lining of the bronchial tubes, this causes long-term cough with mucus, which is chronic bronchitis. Smoking is the main cause of chronic bronchitis and, by extension, the condition is prevalent in people with mental health problems. A systematic review of 114 studies found an elevated risk for chronic bronchitis in those who smoke (Forey *et al.* 2011). Repeatedly breathing in fumes that irritate and damage lung and airway tissues causes chronic bronchitis. Breathing in air pollution and dust or fumes from the environment or workplace also can lead to chronic bronchitis. Viruses or bacteria can easily infect the irritated bronchial tubes and, if this happens, the condition worsens and lasts longer. As a result, people who have chronic bronchitis have periods when symptoms get much worse than usual.

The signs and symptoms of chronic bronchitis include coughing, wheezing and chest discomfort. The coughing may produce large amounts of mucus and we call this smoker's cough. If a patient has chronic bronchitis and COPD it is incumbent to prescribe medicines to open airways and help clear away mucus. These medicines include bronchodilators and steroids. Oxygen therapy is also a useful treatment for chronic bronchitis, as it helps the patient to breathe more easily. An important component of COPD is emphysema and we will turn to this next. But before we do, please take part in the activity below.

Activity 6.4   *Evidence-based practice and research*

Alone or in a group, find out about common household irritants that a patient with chronic bronchitis should avoid.

Emphysema

Emphysema is a result of millions of the lungs' tiny air sacs (alveoli) stretching out of shape or rupturing, which results in the lungs losing their natural elasticity. Emphysema progressively deteriorates over time and the lungs lose their ability to absorb oxygen and release carbon dioxide. Patients' breathing progressively becomes difficult and they are easily short of breath, as if not getting enough air. Emphysema and chronic bronchitis often occur together and are the two most common forms of COPD. Smoking is the main cause of the vast majority of cases of emphysema. Exposure to second-hand smoke and airborne toxins also can contribute to emphysema, though to a much lesser degree. Smokers exposed to high levels of air pollution appear to be at higher risk of developing COPD (Parasuramalu *et al.* 2014).

These respiratory symptoms are the same regardless of the cause of the emphysema. However, two people with the same degree of lung damage may have different symptoms. One person with mild emphysema may feel very short of breath. Another person with more advanced stages of the disease may be hardly bothered by symptoms.

Other symptoms caused by emphysema include:

- wheezing;
- coughing;
- bringing up phlegm (if chronic bronchitis is also present);
- feeling of tightness in the chest;
- barrel-like distended chest;
- constant fatigue;
- difficulty sleeping;
- morning headaches;
- weight loss;
- swelling of the ankles;
- lethargy or difficulty concentrating.

Tertiary prevention of emphysema

If the patient smokes, you should discuss smoking and emphysema with the patient (see Chapter 3). The best way of preventing or slowing down progression of emphysema is to stop smoking (Milot *et al.* 2007). It is also important to advise the patient to limit exposure to air pollution and to restrict outdoor activity when there are reports of high smog levels. Those who experience high exposure to chemicals at work should wear respirator masks or consult with a specialist in occupational medicine. If your patient has emphysema, advise and assist him/her to have a vaccination against influenza (flu) and pneumococcal pneumonia. These vaccinations can help to prevent life-threatening respiratory infections in people with lung disease. The treatment of emphysema cannot reverse symptoms but it can help to relieve symptoms, treat complications and minimise the patient's disability.

Treatment of emphysema

The treatment of emphysema involves the use of bronchodilators to relieve symptoms. Common bronchodilators in use for emphysema are tiotropium, ipratropium, albuterol and salbutamol.

The patient can take the medication in a hand-held inhaler or machine-driven nebuliser. The second group of medicines for emphysema are corticosteroids. These medications help to reduce inflammation in the lungs and during an acute episode of emphysema; we give corticosteroids in tablet or injection form. In the case of acute exacerbation of COPD that is triggered by infection, we use antibiotics for treatment.

For patients whose blood oxygen is below normal, the administration of oxygen therapy can increase life expectancy in people with emphysema. People with emphysema are also at risk of becoming malnourished and you need to discuss and monitor dietary intake with your patient. As we discussed previously, COPD is likely to worsen existing mental health problems and therefore you should be vigilant of this complication and take remedial steps. An improvement in the patient's COPD is likely to promote good mental health and vice versa.

To enhance good health, the patient can take part in pulmonary rehabilitation, a type of physical therapy that teaches the patient to conserve energy, improve stamina and reduce breathlessness.

Another important lung condition is pneumonia and we will discuss this next.

Pneumonia

Pneumonia is an inflammatory condition of the lung affecting primarily the alveoli, which may fill up with fluid or pus. Viruses, bacterial infection and, less commonly, other microorganisms usually cause pneumonia. This condition affects approximately 450 million people globally per year (7% of the population) and results in about 4 million deaths, mostly in developing countries. There is an association between the use of second-generation antipsychotics such as quetiepine, risperidone, clozapine and olanzapine with pneumonia, particularly in the elderly (Trifiro 2011). In a study of patients with mental health problems that spanned over 9 years, the investigators found that those with schizophrenia had a threefold increased risk of the development of pneumonia (Chou *et al.* 2013).

Typical symptoms of pneumonia include a cough, chest pain, fever and difficulty breathing (Figure 6.4). The symptoms of pneumonia can range from mild to severe and many factors influence their severity. These factors are the type of germ causing the infection, the patient's age and overall health.

Pneumonia tends to be more serious in children, people of 65 years or older and those with diabetes, heart failure, COPD and HIV/AIDS. Diabetes and cardiac problems are common in people with mental health problems (see Chapters 4 and 5); therefore by extension, pneumonia is likely to be more serious in this population.

Treatment of pneumonia

For people with mild pneumonia, it is possible to treat this at home by advising the patient to take antibiotics and have plenty of rest and fluids. For those whose pneumonia is due to bacterial infection, you should inform them that they may continue to cough for 2–3 weeks after finishing the antibiotic course and may feel irritable and tired for even longer, as the body continues to recover. To reduce the pain and fever, you may advise the patient to take painkillers such as

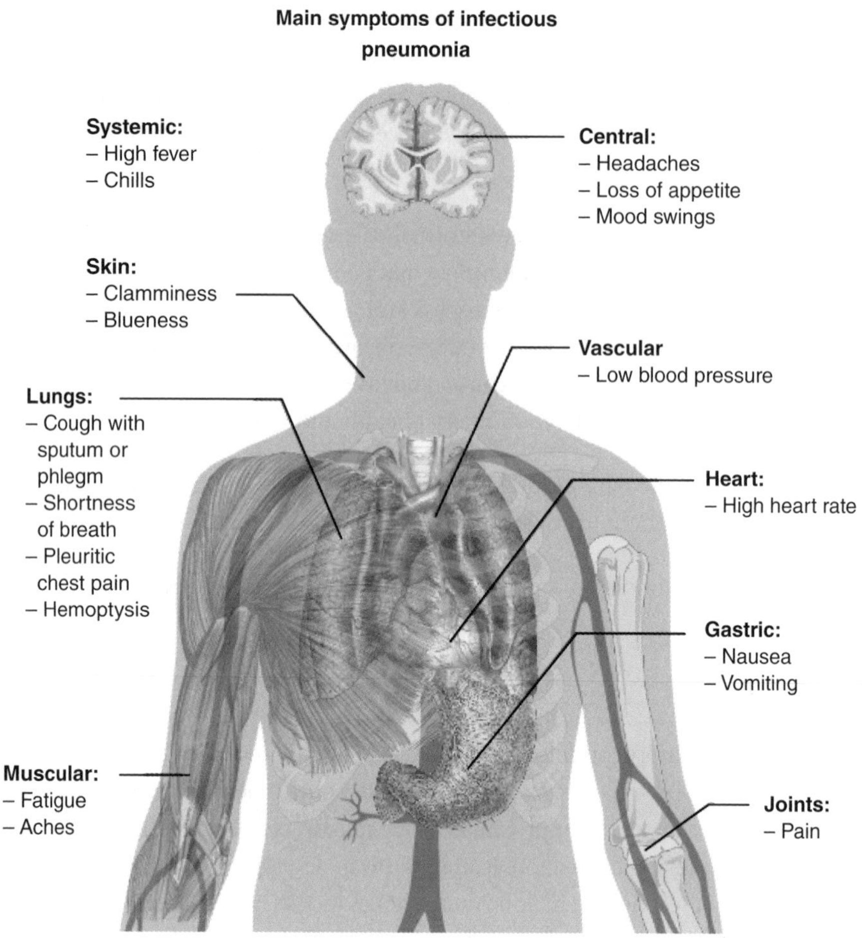

Main symptoms of infectious pneumonia

Systemic:
– High fever
– Chills

Central:
– Headaches
– Loss of appetite
– Mood swings

Skin:
– Clamminess
– Blueness

Vascular
– Low blood pressure

Lungs:
– Cough with
  sputum or
  phlegm
– Shortness
  of breath
– Pleuritic
  chest pain
– Hemoptysis

Heart:
– High heart rate

Gastric:
– Nausea
– Vomiting

Muscular:
– Fatigue
– Aches

Joints:
– Pain

Figure 6.4: Symptoms of pneumonia

paracetamol or ibuprofen. Patients should not take ibuprofen if they are allergic to aspirin or other NSAIDs or have asthma, kidney disease, a history of stomach ulcers or indigestion.

You should advise the patient against the use of cough medicines. Coughing allows mucus to clear from the lungs, so trying to stop coughing could make the pneumonia last even longer. In addition, there is little evidence that cough medicines are effective (Chang *et al.* 2012). You can advise the patient to take a warm drink of honey and lemon to help relieve the discomfort that coughing causes.

Chapter summary

COPD and asthma contribute significantly to global mortality and morbidity. Frequently COPD is comorbid with mental health problems such as depression, anxiety and schizophrenia. In particular, studies have shown a strong association between depression, anxiety, schizophrenia and asthma, suggesting these conditions share a pathophysiological mechanism with asthma. Key treatment for acute asthma is short-acting beta-agonists and inhaled steroids. For uncontrolled chronic asthma, treatment involves the use of LABAs in addition to steroids.

An important element of COPD is bronchitis and this condition is very common in people with mental health problems, mainly because there is a high prevalence of smoking in this population. Treatment for acute bronchitis consists of simple measures such as encouraging the patient to get plenty of rest, drink plenty of fluids and avoid smoke and fumes. For chronic bronchitis, treatment consists of LABAs and steroids.

A second component of COPD is emphysema, which is characterised by inflammation, enlargement and loss of elasticity of the alveoli; thus making gaseous exchange inefficient. As in bronchitis, typical treatment for emphysema is bronchodilators and steroids. If the patient has bacterial infection, then antibiotics are indicated.

Pneumonia is an inflammation of the alveoli, which tend to fill up with pus. This is mainly due to viral, fungal or bacterial infection, and treatment typically involves the use of antibiotics and NSAIDS, to reduce fever.

Activities: Brief outline answers

Activity 6.1

Allergic dermatitis, rhinitis, psoriasis, eczema and urticaria.

Activity 6.2

It is likely that Judy is suffering from stress due to impending exams. Stress is one of the trigger factors for symptoms of asthma. Because Judy's sleep pattern is fractured, this is likely to lower her immune system, making her vulnerable to infection. Infection, particularly of the pulmonary system, is likely to complicate or make the asthma symptoms difficult to control. Also, she is more likely to suffer exacerbation of bipolar disorder due to sleep disturbance.

Activity 6.3

Lack of energy, poor concentration, low mood, cognitive deficits, poor motivation and suicidal ideation can all be symptoms of depression that may interfere with management of asthma.

Activity 6.4

Strong odours or fumes, including household cleaners, perfumes, air fresheners, paints, pet odours and even cooking odours.

Further reading

Cormac I, Gray D (2012) *Essential Physical Health in Psychiatry.* London: Royal College of Psychiatrists.

Nash M (2010) *Physical Health and Wellbeing in Mental Health Nursing: Clinical skills for practice.* Maidenhead, Berkshire: Open University Press.

Useful websites

http://www.nhlbi.nih.gov

This useful website provides information in non-professional language for both service users and professionals about respiratory problems and their management.

https://www.brit-thoracic.org.uk

This website provides information and the latest research information on respiratory conditions.

http://www.who.int/respiratory/copd/en

This website provides worldwide information on the prevalence of COPD and its management.

Chapter 7
Substance misuse and physical health in mental health

NMC Standards for Pre-registration Nursing Education

This chapter will address the following competencies:

Domain 3: Nursing practice and decision-making

Generic standard for competence
All nurses must practise autonomously, compassionately, skilfully and safely, and must maintain dignity and promote health and wellbeing. They must assess and meet the full range of essential physical and mental health needs of people of all ages who come into their care. Where necessary they must be able to provide safe and effective immediate care to all people prior to accessing or referring to specialist services irrespective of their field of practice. All nurses must also meet more complex and coexisting needs for people in their own nursing field of practice, in any setting including hospital, community and at home. All practice should be informed by the best available evidence and comply with local and national guidelines. Decision-making must be shared with service users, carers and families and informed by critical analysis of a full range of possible interventions, including the use of up-to-date technology. All nurses must also understand how behaviour, culture, socioeconomic and other factors, in the care environment and its location, can affect health, illness, health outcomes and public health priorities and take this into account in planning and delivering care.

NMC Essential Skills Clusters

This chapter will address the following ESCs:

1. People can trust the newly registered graduate nurse to provide care based on the highest standards, knowledge and competence.
2. People can trust the newly registered graduate nurse to engage them as partners in care.
6. People can trust the newly registered graduate nurse to listen and provide information that is clear, accurate and meaningful at a level at which the patient/client can understand.
9. People can trust the newly registered graduate nurse to treat them as partners and work with them to make a holistic and systematic assessment of their needs; to develop a personalised plan that is based on mutual understanding and respect for their individual situation promoting health and well-being, minimising risk of harm and promoting their safety at all times.

Introduction

Case study

Tony is a 27-year-old male who suffers from bipolar disorder. He has been taking drugs and alcohol since he was a teenager. In addition to abusing alcohol, marijuana and crack cocaine, he smokes 30 cigarettes a day. He has sold drugs in the past and has several convictions for supplying drugs. After a binge on amphetamines and alcohol he became so depressed that he attempted suicide. He was admitted to the psychiatric wing of his local hospital. After 6 weeks in hospital, Tony recovered and resolved to give up drugs and alcohol.

Substance misuse is defined as the harmful use of substances like drugs and alcohol for non-medical purposes. It occurs when individuals continue to find and use substances to alter their mind even if these substances cause serious harmful effects to themselves or others. The term substance misuse often refers to illegal drugs but can also include legal substances like alcohol, prescription medications, caffeine, nicotine and volatiles.

Millions of people worldwide misuse substances each year and this has profound consequences for their health, as in Tony's case. Each year, approximately 76.3 million people struggle with alcohol use disorders, contributing to 1.8 million deaths per year (WHO 2014b). Approximately 40% of patients with mental health problems also use substances such as alcohol, illicit drugs or nicotine (Munro and Edward 2008). Like Tony, people with mental health problems may misuse more than one substance. Several studies have found a link between the use of substances and mental health (see Chapter 1). Critically, there is a clear association between the misuse of cannabis and psychosis, especially in those who present with an early onset of psychosis. In other words, the misuse of substances can expose an individual to psychotic illness at an earlier age (Farrelly *et al.* 2007). The misuse can occur at any phase of the patient's illness and this usually includes multiple patterns of use and non-use.

Because of the complex nature of substance misuse and its accompanying social and health consequences, it is difficult to offer a single causal explanation that applies to all individuals in all cultures. However, popular theories suggest that the use of substances is a form of self-medication, a genetic vulnerability, environment or lifestyle. At one end of the spectrum, it is possible to view substance misuse as criminal conduct, a moral failing or evidence of the individual's social incompatibility. On the other end of the spectrum, we consider the problematic use of substances as a bio-behavioural act driven by an individual's genetic makeup. For example, some investigators estimate that up to 70% of the **variance** we associate with drug abuse or dependence is genetically heritable (Kendler *et al.* 2007). Apart from these two polar views, there is a general acceptance that environmental factors play an enormously powerful role in the development and continuation of problematic substance use, especially as they interact with particular individual characteristics (Sloboda *et al.* 2012). Irrespective of the aetiology of substance misuse, there is a clear neurobiological pathway responsible for the behaviour we see in many people with such problems. However, before we discuss these, let us think about the consequences of substance abuse.

Activity 7.1 **Critical thinking**

Alone or in a group, make a list of the various consequences of abusing substances to the person, family and to the treatment process.

There are outline answers to all the activities at the end of the chapter.

The dopamine theory of reward

In psychology, a reward is any process that reinforces behaviour. In other words, it is something that, when offered, causes a behaviour to increase in intensity. In addition, rewards induce

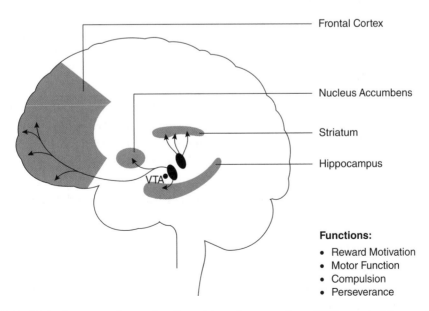

Figure 7.1: Critical neuropathways implicated in substance abuse. VTA, ventral tegmental area

learning and feelings of positive emotions and natural rewards; examples of rewards are eating, drinking, sex and fighting.

There is the general acceptance that the reward circuit, or the dopamine mesolimbic system, is the common pathway of reward and reinforcement in people with substance misuse disorder. We refer to this pathway as the 'pleasure centre' and within it dopamine is the 'pleasure neurotransmitter'. It is a very old pathway from an evolutionary point of view and the use of dopamine neurons to control behavioural responses to natural rewards is present even in worms and flies, which evolved 1–2 billion years ago. An increase in dopamine levels in the mesolimbic system (reward system) produces a pleasurable feeling and there are many natural ways to trigger release of dopamine in the mesolimbic system. The mesolimbic system includes the dopamine-containing neurons of the ventral tegmental area, the nucleus accumbens and part of the prefrontal cortex (Figure 7.1). The pleasure we experience when passing an examination, listening to music we enjoy, watching a funny movie, eating food, drinking, sex, and so on, is a result of dopamine release in these regions. By contrast, there is a depression of dopamine neurons when there is an omission of the expected reward. In other words, there is no release of dopamine in the reward pathway. In nature, we learn to repeat behaviours that lead to maximising rewards. Thus, we learn to repeat behaviours that lead to an increase in dopamine in the reward system. To be able to produce these feelings of joy or 'natural highs' there is an array of chemicals that regulate dopamine in the mesolimbic pathway and these include the brain's own natural drugs like endorphins, opiates, anandamide (cannabis) and acetylcholine (nicotine).

Nearly all substances of abuse directly or indirectly target the brain's reward system by flooding the circuit with dopamine. The overstimulation of this system that normally responds to natural behaviours such as eating, drinking and listening to music produces euphoric effects. When an individual takes substances of abuse like drugs, the release of dopamine in the reward system can be up to ten times the amount that natural rewards release, thus dwarfing natural reward production. In some cases, this release occurs almost immediately, as in intravenous injection or smoking of drugs. Further, the effects can last for much longer than those of natural rewards. Such a powerful reward strongly motivates people to take drugs repeatedly and therefore this reaction sets in motion a pattern that 'teaches' people to repeat the behaviour of abusing these substances.

Tolerance and addiction

As a person continues to abuse substances, the brain responds by adapting to the overwhelming surges in dopamine, producing less dopamine or reducing the number of dopamine receptors in the reward circuit. This lessens the impact of dopamine on the reward circuit, therefore reducing the abuser's ability to enjoy the substances. Individuals may now require larger amounts of the drug than they first did to achieve the original dopamine high, and we call this effect *tolerance*. Users may resort to committing crime to finance a substance abuse habit and this brings them in conflict with law enforcement agencies.

Substances of abuse facilitate non-conscious (conditioned) learning, which leads users to experience uncontrollable cravings when they see a place or person they associate with the drug experience, even when the drug itself is not available. Brain imaging studies of drug-addicted individuals show changes in areas of the brain that are critical to judgement, decision making, learning and memory, and behaviour control. Together, these changes can drive abusers to seek out and take substances compulsively despite adverse consequences. In other words, they become addicted to drugs. In particular, alcohol can cause profound health consequences but before we discuss this, let's think about our own response to these processes.

> ### Scenario
>
> *You receive a phone call from one of your patients who drinks heavily, informing you that he wishes to 'end it all'. He has not been drinking for a day and feels irritable and sweaty. He is not sure whether he should continue to drink alcohol or not and he needs help to 'sort his life out'. How would you respond to this call?*

The first thing you should do is to go and see your patient as a matter of urgency. Check his level of commitment to give up drinking. The fact that he has called for you is an indication that he has made some sort of commitment to giving up but he may be unsure. You should explore this ambivalence with him and offer information, particularly on his treatment options. Offer detoxification if possible, probably as an inpatient because abruptly stopping drinking can have serious health risks. You will need to contact the doctor and arrange for hospital admission if possible.

Alcohol

The production and use of alcoholic beverages is common in many cultures and may go as far back as the Egyptian and Mesopotamian civilisations. In many parts of the world, drinking alcoholic beverages is a common feature of social gatherings. Because alcohol is legal and is integral to the socialisation process in many cultures, it is not seen as a drug or harmful to our health. Nevertheless, alcohol is intoxicating, toxic and dependence producing, and its consumption carries a risk of adverse health and social consequences. The harmful use of alcohol is a global problem which compromises both individual and social development. It results in 2.5 million deaths each year (WHO 2011d). Alcohol is the world's third largest risk factor for premature mortality, disability and loss of health; it is the leading risk factor in the western world. The use of alcohol has an association with many serious social and developmental issues, including violence, child abuse and absenteeism in the workplace. It also causes harm far beyond the physical and psychological health of the drinker. It harms the well-being and health of people around the drinker. Intoxicated indidivuals can harm others or put them at risk of traffic accidents and violent behaviour; they can negatively affect co-workers, relatives, friends or strangers. Thus, the impact of the harmful use of alcohol reaches deep into society.

In the UK, about 23% of the adult population drink alcohol in a hazardous or harmful way (Drummond 2004). Estimates are that 38% of men and 16% of women aged 16–64 in the UK consume more alcohol than the recommended sensible limit. The annual cost of alcohol-related crime and public disorder in the UK approximates £7.3 billion, workplace costs are up to £6.4 billion and healthcare costs are £1.4–1.7 billion per year. As well as this very significant public cost,

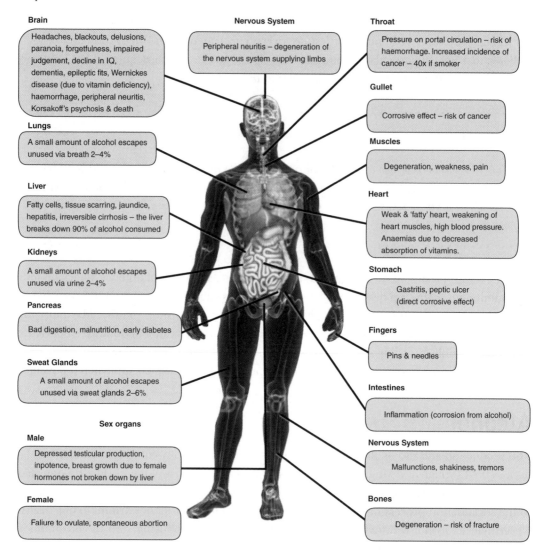

Brain
Headaches, blackouts, delusions, paranoia, forgetfulness, impaired judgement, decline in IQ, dementia, epileptic fits, Wernickes disease (due to vitamin deficiency), haemorrhage, peripheral neuritis, Korsakoff's psychosis & death

Lungs
A small amount of alcohol escapes unused via breath 2–4%

Liver
Fatty cells, tissue scarring, jaundice, hepatitis, irreversible cirrhosis – the liver breaks down 90% of alcohol consumed

Kidneys
A small amount of alcohol escapes unused via urine 2–4%

Pancreas
Bad digestion, malnutrition, early diabetes

Sweat Glands
A small amount of alcohol escapes unused via sweat glands 2–6%

Sex organs
Male
Depressed testicular production, inpotence, breast growth due to female hormones not broken down by liver

Female
Faliure to ovulate, spontaneous abortion

Nervous System
Peripheral neuritis – degeneration of the nervous system supplying limbs

Throat
Pressure on portal circulation – risk of haemorrhage. Increased incidence of cancer – 40x if smoker

Gullet
Corrosive effect – risk of cancer

Muscles
Degeneration, weakness, pain

Heart
Weak & 'fatty' heart, weakening of heart muscles, high blood pressure. Anaemias due to decreased absorption of vitamins.

Stomach
Gastritis, peptic ulcer (direct corrosive effect)

Fingers
Pins & needles

Intestines
Inflammation (corrosion from alcohol)

Nervous System
Malfunctions, shakiness, tremors

Bones
Degeneration – risk of fracture

Figure 7.2: Disorders that alcohol can cause. (Reproduced with permission from http://www. alcoholservices-ateam.org.uk/effects_of_alcohol.html © The Rehabilitation for Addicted Prisoners Trust (RAPt) and Peter Gould.)

there are direct effects on the individual, with alcohol causing around 60 different types of diseases and medical conditions (Anderson and Baumberg 2006). Some of these are shown in Figure 7.2.

A weekly alcohol consumption of 22–50 units for men and 15–35 units for women is likely to increase an individual's risk of developing alcohol-related harm. The World Health Organization (WHO) defines harmful drinking as a state *where there is clear evidence that alcohol is contributing substantially to physical or psychological harm, including impaired judgement or dysfunctional behaviour which may lead to disability or have an adverse consequence for interpersonal relationships* (WHO 1992).

Blood alcohol levels

Binge drinking can lead to a fast increase in blood alcohol concentration and consequently to drunkenness. In adults who do not drink regularly, relatively low blood alcohol levels

(50–150 mg/dL) result in intoxication that includes the following symptoms: impaired sense of time and space, poor coordination, reduction in reaction times, poor concentration, memory difficulties, impairment of judgement, pinpoint pupils and red eyes (conjunctival injection). Severe intoxication (300–500 mg/dL) has an association with further deterioration in these symptoms. Alcohol depresses the vital centres in the central nervous system, which may lead to hypotension, stupor, respiratory failure and cardiac arrest, leading to death. Cardiac arrhythmia is another potentially fatal complication of an alcohol binge.

We move now to look at the long-term effects of alcohol consumption on other organ systems.

Effects of long-term alcohol misuse

Alcohol is the most common cause of liver injury in high-income countries; deaths due to cirrhosis of the liver are rising at an increasing rate in the UK. This contrasts with the rest of western Europe, where corresponding mortality rates are decreasing (Leon and McCambridge 2006). Alcohol causes three types of liver disorders: fatty liver or steatosis, alcoholic hepatitis and cirrhosis. Fatty liver is the accumulation of triglycerides in the liver cells (hepatocytes). Its prognosis is benign so long as patients abstain from alcohol. However, up to 30% of patients who continue to drink progress to cirrhosis within 10 years.

The key features of alcoholic hepatitis are fatty liver, liver cell damage, a neutrophil infiltrate and **pericellular fibrosis**. Presentation can be asymptomatic, but severe alcoholic hepatitis often presents with painless jaundice on the background of heavy alcohol consumption.

Cirrhosis

A typical characteristic of liver cirrhosis is the replacement of liver tissue with scar tissue (fibrosis) and **regenerative nodules**. These changes lead to loss of liver function. Up to 90% of deaths in patients with alcoholic cirrhosis have a direct link with the liver.

The gastrointestinal tract

Although mortality from alcohol-related gastrointestinal effects is low, morbidity is high. The toxic effects of long-term alcohol misuse are due to nutritional deficiencies (Kaludjerovic and Vieth 2010). These can cause **stomatitis** and **glossitis**, where there may be a reduction in salivary production. Further, there may be chronic inflammation of the mucosa of the mouth and pharynx, resulting in pre-cancerous lesions we call leukoplakia, erythroplakia and submucous fibrosis. Nausea and vomiting are common features of alcohol misuse and may induce **Mallory–Weiss tears**. This is a syndrome caused by a tear in the lining of the upper part of the gastrointestinal tract. The tear causes bleeding and other symptoms. Gastritis and duodenitis can both result from alcohol misuse.

Alcohol abuse causes vitamin deficiencies and the most common are deficiencies of thiamine, niacin and vitamin C. This results in Wernicke–Korsakoff syndrome and beri-beri (typically dry) pellagra, and symptoms of scurvy respectively. Alcohol is second only to biliary disease as a leading cause of acute and chronic pancreatitis.

The cardiovascular system

Almost 50% of the excess deaths due to alcohol misuse are attributable to circulatory disease rather than to liver disease. Alcohol is a common cause of both systolic and diastolic hypertension. Additionally, there is an association between all types of stroke and binge drinking. Long-term, heavy alcohol consumption is the main cause of a non-ischaemic, dilated cardiomyopathy and increases the risk of cardiac arrhythmias regardless of the presence of heart disease. In contrast, drinking alcohol in moderation has a protective effect on the cardiovascular system, but when the consumption is greater than 2.5 units per day, alcohol increases the risk for cardiovascular disease.

The respiratory system

At high doses, alcohol decreases respiratory rate, airflow and oxygen transport, so it worsens many symptoms of pulmonary disease. One of the most serious complications of alcohol binges is aspiration pneumonia. The depressant effects of alcohol are via its activating effect on the inhibitory neurotransmitter gamma-aminobutyric acid (GABA). Alcohol enhances the inhibitory effect of GABA at its receptor site and at levels above 300 mg/dL it can cause death from respiratory depression (Nutt 1999). Alcohol also inhibits the glutamate receptor, N-methyl-D-aspartate (Hallak *et al.* 2011), at blood levels above 100 mg/dL system, and this adds to its central nervous system-depressant effect.

Alcohol reduces key pulmonary defences against infection, including **mucociliary** clearance: the mobilisation, killing and clearance of macrophages and **phospholipid** metabolism. In chronic heavy drinkers, these actions directly contribute to the increase in rates of pulmonary infection. Long-term alcohol misuse has an association with worsening of acute respiratory distress syndrome.

The nervous system

Alcohol abuse has an association with a wide range of effects on the nervous system. It produces the metabolite acetaldehyde that is directly neurotoxic. More importantly, chronic alcohol abusers tend to suffer nutritional deficiencies which undoubtedly contribute significantly to most alcohol-related neurological diseases (Butterworth 1995). These neurological diseases include neurotoxicity, alcohol dependence syndrome, alcohol withdrawal syndrome, seizures and cognitive deterioration leading to Korsakoff's psychosis, **Wernicke's encephalopathy** and **Wernicke–Korsakoff** syndrome, progressive cerebellar degeneration, acute confusional state, peripheral neuropathy and autonomic neuropathy. Clearly, a chronic misuse of alcohol can worsen psychotic and depressive symptoms. It can also have a negative effect on the endocrine system.

The endocrine system

Alcohol down-regulates the pituitary–gonadal axis, resulting in a reduction of luteinising hormone and follicle-stimulating hormone serum levels, causing shrinkage of the sex glands (gonads). Overall, this reduces the serum levels of sex hormones, causing reduction in libido, impotence, menstrual irregularities and infertility.

Long-term, heavy alcohol misuse activates the hypothalamus–pituitary–adrenal (HPA) axis. Alcohol withdrawal induces physiological and psychological stress which in turn increases HPA activity. High HPA activity causes unstable levels of corticotrophin-releasing factor (CRF) and cortisol. CRF is a key chemical for initiating many of the endocrine, autonomic and behavioural responses to stress. Cortisol is a hormone that helps to maintain blood pressure, immune function and the body's anti-inflammatory processes. An increase in CRF and cortisol induces various pathological states, including pseudo-Cushing's syndrome, osteoporosis, diabetes mellitus, depression and hypertension as well as impairment in immune function and alcohol withdrawal seizures.

The misuse of alcohol also interferes with the metabolism of glucose.

Glucose metabolism

In the long term, glucose intolerance (pre-diabetes) is common in those who misuse alcohol. Alcohol and its metabolite acetaldehyde stop or reduce the secretion of insulin in a dose-dependent manner. Thus, the more alcohol the person drinks, the more likely s/he is to develop glucose intolerance. Other detrimental effects of alcohol on glucose metabolism are increases in corticosteroids and ketoacidosis, as well as altered levels of circulating dopamine, noradrenaline and adrenaline.

Although low alcohol consumption has a protective effect against type 2 diabetes, higher consumption increases the risk of developing the disorder. This is because at low doses (10–20 g/day) alcohol increases insulin sensitivity, but at higher doses it has a harmful effect on carbohydrate metabolism, including insulin resistance (Hodge *et al.* 2006). Other endocrine abnormalities include obesity, sodium retention and low levels of parathyroid hormone, magnesium and calcium. Chronic alcohol misuse is a risk factor for the development of osteoporosis.

Other effects

Chronic alcohol consumption can cause various skin disorders, including psoriasis, discoid eczema and basal cell carcinomas. Its long-term misuse has an association with water and salt retention, causing an expanded extracellular volume and impairment of the kidneys. Heavy alcohol consumption has an association with various cancers, particularly of the upper alimentary tract, liver, colon, rectum and breast. Among other mechanisms, alcohol usage can cause cancers by altering blood hormone levels, especially causing an elevation in oestrogen-related hormones, which may increase the risk of breast cancer through increases in cell growth and alterations (Oyesanmi *et al.* 2010). It is therefore important that you should discuss the harmful effects of alcohol with your patient.

Acute treatment of alcohol withdrawal

Case study

Bethany is a 43-year-old woman who was diagnosed with bipolar disorder 20 years ago. She was found lying unconscious across her front door by her community psychiatric nurse (CPN). All the indications suggested Bethany had taken an overdose of an unknown quantity of whisky and sodium valproate.

continued . . .

> *The nurse saw a short note written by Bethany suggesting that she could no longer cope with the ravages of bipolar disorder and alcohol.*
>
> *The CPN phoned for the ambulance straight away and, whilst she was waiting for the ambulance to arrive, she ensured Bethany had a clear airway and recorded pulse and respiration until the ambulance arrived 6 minutes later. The CPN put the empty bottles of whisky and sodium valproate in a bag for the ambulance crew to take with them.*
>
> *Bethany was taken to hospital where a gastric lavage was performed. After staying in hospital for 2 days, she was transferred to the psychiatric wing where she received treatment for 4 weeks. During her stay in hospital, she felt sufficiently supported and motivated to give up alcohol. She was subsequently discharged with an agreed care package that focused on assisting her to give up alcohol.*

Management of alcohol misuse

Your first responsibility as a nurse is to bring patients to a point of readiness to change their substance misuse behaviour by applying the popular 'stages of change' model (Prochaska and DiClemente 1984). This means that the patient has to reach at least the contemplation stage (see Chapter 3), as in the case of Bethany. At this stage, patients are sufficiently well motivated to make a sustained effort to change. In other words, they have reached a good-quality decision to change not because they are under pressure from family or work, or because they simply feel the need for a temporary break from drinking. In the case of Bethany, circumstances surrounding her being found suggest she clearly is desperate to give up alcohol.

Your patient needs accurate information about what to expect during detoxification as information is likely to reduce the severity of the withdrawal and increase adherence (Phillips *et al.* 1986). In the course of discussion with the patient, map out a timetable for the week in which detoxification will take place and for the following week, as it will bring up a number of important issues. In Bethany's case, the discussion should happen before she goes to the psychiatric wing of the hospital.

During the discussion, work out and assist the patient with practical concerns. For example, organising time off work, if the patient is working, and meeting any childcare responsibilities. If the patient is travelling to an outpatient unit daily, are there any transport difficulties? If the patient has pets, are arrangements in place for their care? Is there someone who is willing to support the patient through the first week of detoxification?

Before detoxification, you should provide a good assessment that is thorough and comprehensive, with the purpose of identifying the person's nature and severity of any substance misuse-related problem. In addition, a full physical assessment is necessary. In Bethany's case, this should include any ill effects she may have suffered from the sodium valproate overdose.

It is important to understand the cause of the problem and to assess its consequences in order to establish the patient's strengths and weaknesses. Bethany drinks mainly as a way of managing the symptoms of her bipolar disorder. If you carry out a good assessment, you will be able to formulate an overall care plan that is the basis of good care. As with any care, the plan should have a good evidence base, including harm reduction approaches (Department of Health 2007).

Another aspect that promotes good care is effective key working.

Effective key working

The National Institute for Health and Care Excellence (NICE) guidelines (National Clinical Guidelines Centre 2010) stipulate that effective key working is an important element of treatment and care. It helps to deliver high-quality outcomes for people who misuse substances. If you are a key worker, you have a central role in coordinating a care plan and building a therapeutic alliance with the patient. The benefits of any treatment approach in substance misuse can only be realised within this context. You must also take into account the patient's needs and preferences. People who misuse substances should have the opportunity to make informed decisions about their care and treatment, in partnership with you. If a patient does not have the capacity to make decisions, you should let the Mental Capacity Act 2005 guide you in your decision making. You should support any information you give to the patient with evidence.

As with any intervention, the information you give to patients regarding their treatment should have a credible evidence base, specific to the patient's needs and culturally appropriate. Always ensure that any information you give is accessible to people with additional needs, such as sensory or learning disabilities, and to people who do not speak or read English (Mutsatsa 2011). If the patient agrees, you should involve families and carers in decisions regarding care and management. You should also give them the information and support they need. The first stage in the care of people with alcohol misuse problems is detoxification, and we will now look at this in more detail.

Alcohol detoxification

Alcohol withdrawal syndrome is an uncommon but potentially life-threatening condition affecting some alcohol-dependent patients who suddenly discontinue or decrease their alcohol consumption. In general, less than half of alcoholic patients report withdrawal symptoms. In most cases, these symptoms do not require intervention, often disappearing within 2–7 days of the last drink. You should consider inpatient alcohol detoxification if the person:

- is severely dependent on alcohol;
- has a history of delirium tremens and alcohol withdrawal seizures;
- has a poor social support network;
- has poor physical health that includes cardiac, pulmonary, hepatic, kidney or cardiovascular diseases;
- has cognitive and memory impairment;
- has psychiatric comorbidity (e.g. depression, psychosis or personality disorder).

You should be aware that the manifestation of alcohol withdrawal tends to differ from person to person but usually occurs within 6–24 hours after the last drink. Symptoms include mild insomnia, increase in blood pressure and pulse rate, tremors, **hyper-reflexia**, irritability, anxiety and depression in some people.

The symptoms of severe alcohol withdrawal syndrome may progress to a more complex form with characteristic features of delirium tremens, seizures and coma. In these forms, cardiac arrest and death may occur in 5–10% of patients (Schuckit *et al.* 1995). For this reason, it is important for you to assess the level or severity of dependency in an individual, preferably using a clinical rating scale. There are many rating scales for assessment of alcohol withdrawal: the best-known and most extensively studied scale is the Clinical Institute Withdrawal Assessment – Alcohol (CIWA–A) and a shortened version, the CIWA–A revised (CIWA–Ar). This scale has well-documented reliability based on comparison to ratings by expert clinicians (Wiehl *et al.* 1994). It is easy to use in a variety of clinical settings. The CIWA–Ar has added usefulness because high scores, in addition to indicating severe withdrawal, are also predictive of the development of seizures and delirium. The scale has ten items and each item scores a minimum of 0 and maximum of 7 (Table 7.1).

Total scores on the CIWA of less than 10 indicate minimal to mild withdrawal. Scores of 8–15 indicate moderate withdrawal (marked autonomic arousal); scores of 15 or more indicate severe withdrawal. The assessment can take 2 minutes to complete. A study of the revised version of the CIWA predicted that those with a score of over 15 were at increased risk for severe alcohol withdrawal, thus the higher the score the greater the risk. However, you should be aware that without treatment some patients could suffer complications despite low scores. You should always explain procedures fully to the patient and answer any questions. As usual, always seek consent before carrying out procedures. After assessment, detoxification usually follows and it is to that procedure we will now turn.

Symptom severity	0	1	2	3	4	5	6	7
Agitation								
Anxiety								
Auditory disturbances								
Clouding of sensorium								
Headache								
Nausea/vomiting								
Paroxysmal sweats								
Tactile disturbances								
Tremor								
Visual disturbances								

Table 7.1: The Clinical Institute Withdrawal Assessment – Alcohol revised (CIWA–Ar) scale

Detoxification procedure

The process of alcohol detoxification requires the elimination of alcohol from the body. It also involves the elimination of any physical or psychological withdrawal symptoms. You should be aware that alcohol withdrawal symptoms can be very distressing and can be fatal if the addiction to alcohol is very severe. Some patients, for example Bethany in the case study, need to be under constant supervision as an inpatient for at least a week. This is because sudden cessation of alcohol consumption can lead to other symptoms that require medical intervention. Some patients who undergo the alcohol detoxification process may suffer from hallucinations, delirium tremens and even convulsions, which, if not immediately attended to, can be fatal.

Detoxification regime

You should start by completing a CIWA on admission to the ward, repeated 8-hourly for 24 hours. Record vital signs such as blood pressure, pulse, temperature, oxygen concentration and peak flow. On admission determine blood alcohol concentration using a breathalyser.

Keep recording vital signs every 4 hours and call the doctor if the patient's diastolic blood pressure is greater than 120 mmHg, or systolic blood pressure is greater than 180 mmHg.

At present, benzodiazepines are the medicines of choice in the treatment of alcohol withdrawal as they have proven their efficacy in ameliorating symptoms and decreasing the risk of seizures and delirium tremens. We administer benzodiazepines for the first 7 days. We need to control and monitor drug use properly to ensure that we quickly treat side effects when they occur. An initial dosage is always high, but there is a gradual reduction in dose over the week, which is how long the alcohol detoxification programme generally lasts. Lorazepam and oxazepam are appropriate for patients with liver disease and we use longer-acting ones like chlordiazepoxide for patients with satisfactory health (Mutsatsa 2011).

Dietary needs

People who misuse alcohol are likely to need more nutrients than the general population, firstly because they may substitute alcohol for food. Second, alcohol speeds up the metabolism of essential vitamin nutrients like thiamine and riboflavin so it is important to supplement these nutrients as they assist with blood circulation and glucose metabolism. Cerebral beri-beri or Wernicke's encephalopathy is a common complication of thiamine (vitamin B_1) deficiency, and to avoid this we normally give thiamine for about 5 days, followed by oral vitamin-B compound. Patients with extreme alcohol withdrawal syndrome need thiamine injection as oral thiamine is poorly absorbed in those who have been drinking heavily. Long-term alcohol abusers are likely to have a deficiency of folic acid. Therefore, supplementing this nutrient (800–1,000 µg/day) is important.

Most of the toxic effects of alcohol are a result of the production of free radicals such as aldehydes. It is important that the patient eats food rich in vitamins A, C and E and beta-carotene as they act as antioxidants that clean up free radicals. Food rich in antioxidants are carrots, squash, broccoli, sweet potatoes, tomatoes, mangoes, oranges, sweet lime, green peppers, green leafy vegetables, blackcurrants, whole grains, green leafy vegetables, kiwi fruit, vegetable oil and fish-liver oil. Other important dietary intakes for people with alcohol abuse are zinc, calcium, essential fatty acids and glutathione (see Chapter 9).

Activity 7.2   *Critical thinking*

You have been asked to carry out admission procedures on a 45-year-old man who suffers from depression. During the admission interview, he appears irritable, forgetful and shows fine tremors. He informs you that he has been drinking two bottles of whisky a day. In light of this new information, what might you incorporate in the admission procedure?

Long-term relapse prevention

The long-term care of people with alcohol misuse problems should be carried out in the community, and medicines play a small part. You should note that the use of medicines to treat substance-related problems without psychosocial intervention sends the wrong message to the patient. The substance abuser already leans heavily on substances either to escape or solve problems and we should not collude in the dependence on substances to solve all problems. Nevertheless, medicines do play an important role in the recovery journey of the patient.

Several medicines have been licensed for the long-term treatment of alcohol dependence. Medicines such as naltrexone work by blocking opioid receptors, therefore limiting dopamine's release into the reward system. By limiting the amount of dopamine in the reward system, the medicine naltrexone effectively blocks the enjoyment of drinking. Another long-term pharmacological treatment of alcohol dependence is aversion therapy.

In aversion therapy, the medication will make the effects of using alcohol extremely uncomfortable. Based on the aversion therapy principle, the medicine disulfiram discourages the patient from drinking by producing an adverse reaction when the patient takes alcohol but has minimal effects when a person abstains. A third and popular method for the treatment of long-term alcohol misuse involves the use of the medicine acamprosate. Because withdrawal of alcohol following chronic usage can lead to excessive glutamate activity and a reduction in GABA activity, acamprosate appears to work by stimulating the GABA receptors and decreases excitation at the glutamate receptors (Hallak *et al.* 2011). It can suppress alcohol-induced dopamine increase in the nucleus accumbens part of the reward system.

Tobacco smoking

Case study

Jacob is a 27-year-old male who suffers from obsessive compulsive disorder. He has been smoking since the age of 16. He has tried to give up several times but has been unsuccessful. He now smokes 35 cigarettes

---

a day and, because he is unemployed, he finds the smoking habit expensive. Although he used to be very active as a teenager (playing rugby and cricket), he runs out of breath very easily and coughs a lot at night. He would like to give up smoking completely; however, he is unsure as to how to proceed.

According to the WHO (2005), tobacco smoking is one of the biggest public health threats the world has ever faced, killing nearly 6 million people a year, and this figure is likely to increase to 8 million a year by 2030. Jacob in the case study is a typical example. More than 5 million of those deaths are the direct result of tobacco use, while more than 600,000 are the result of exposure to second-hand smoke by non-smokers. One person dies approximately every 6 seconds due to tobacco, accounting for one in ten adult deaths. Up to half of current users will eventually die from a tobacco-related disease.

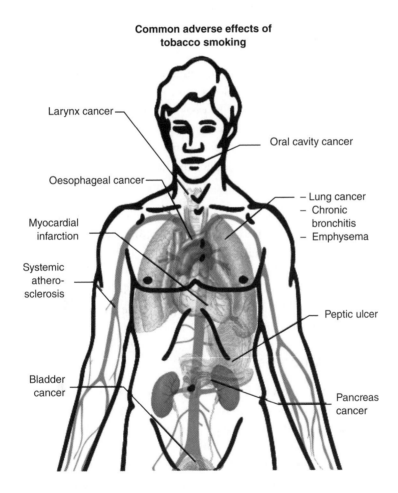

Figure 7.3: The harmful effects of tobacco smoking on body systems and organs. (Reproduced from Häggström M (2014) Medical gallery of Mikael Häggström 2014. Wikiversity Journal of Medicine)

Nearly 800 million smokers worldwide live in low- and middle-income countries, where the burden of tobacco-related illness and death is heaviest. Tobacco users tend to die prematurely, depriving their families of income, raising the cost of healthcare and hindering economic development. Tobacco contains more than 4,000 chemicals, of which at least 250 are harmful to health and more than 50 are carcinogenic (Cancer Research UK).

In the UK, approximately 10 million adults (like Jacob in the case study) smoke tobacco. Over 100,000 smokers in the UK die from smoking-related causes, making it the single most common preventable cause of death in Britain. Smoking accounts for over one-third of respiratory deaths, over one-quarter of cancer deaths and about one-seventh of cardiovascular disease deaths. In general, smoking harms almost every organ of the body (Figure 7.3).

Tobacco smoking is costly in financial terms and the total amount spent on tobacco in the UK in 2011 was estimated at approximately £18.3 billion (The Health and Social Care Information Centre 2012). Smokers pay with their lives, losing on average 8 years compared to non-smokers. A relatively recent study found that those with mental health problems are likely to smoke but less likely to stop smoking than the general population (Smith *et al.* 2014).

Nicotine dependence

Early studies show that tobacco use has a clear dependence potential and people show clear symptoms of withdrawal. These symptoms develop within 12 hours and can persist for 3 weeks, though appetite is increased and can last over 10 weeks (Benowitz 1988). To an extent, these symptoms are experienced after withdrawal of nicotine replacement therapy (NRT), suggesting that they represent a physiological withdrawal from nicotine rather than a behavioural response to the cigarette-smoking process. You need to understand how nicotine produces addiction and influences smoking behaviour in order to provide the best smoking cessation intervention.

When a person inhales tobacco smoke, the lungs absorb the nicotine rapidly into the blood stream. It eventually reaches the brain, where it binds to nicotinic acetylcholine receptors. The binding of nicotine to these receptors acutely increases activity in the prefrontal cortex, thalamus and visual system. The stimulation of these brain regions results in the release of various neurotransmitters, including noradrenaline, acetylcholine, serotonin, GABA, glutamate, endorphins and dopamine. In turn, the release of dopamine in the mesolimbic area (reward system) results in a pleasurable feeling that smokers experience.

The effects of nicotine withdrawal

Smokers come to use nicotine to adjust their level of arousal and for mood control in daily life. Tobacco smoking may improve concentration, reaction time and performance of certain tasks. When a person stops smoking, nicotine withdrawal symptoms emerge (Benowitz 2009). These include irritability, depressed mood, restlessness, anxiety, problems getting along with friends and family, difficulty concentrating, increased hunger and eating, insomnia and craving for tobacco. Nicotine withdrawal can produce mood disturbances comparable in intensity to those seen in psychiatric outpatients with depression (Hughes 2006). For this reason, smokers with depression would benefit from closer monitoring following smoking cessation.

When patients decide to give up smoking, you should discuss this with them. As in alcohol dependence, you want to assist the patient to come to a point of readiness to give up smoking (see Chapter 3). The gold standard for help with smoking cessation is pharmacotherapy plus individual or group specialist behavioural support. This increases fourfold the chances of an individual giving up smoking.

Nicotine replacement therapy

There are several forms of NRT currently available in the UK. These products vary in their speed of nicotine delivery. Combining a nicotine patch with a rapid-delivery form of NRT is more effective than a single type of nicotine replacement. Overall, all commercially available forms of NRT (gum, transdermal patch, nasal spray, inhaler and sublingual tablets/lozenges) can help people to give up smoking and increase their chances of doing so by up to 70% (Stead *et al.* 2012). Moreover, the use of nicotine patches had an association with greater positive mood over time in comparison with nicotine gum in a study of 335 smokers (Strasser *et al.* 2005). This is further supported by a systematic review that concluded that nicotine gum reduces total withdrawal discomfort, irritability and anxiety, and has some positive effect on depressed mood and craving (West and Shiffman 2001).

In those with schizophrenia, evidence suggests that NRT is effective, although not as effective as it is for the general population. There is some evidence that the rapid nicotine delivery of a nasal spray is most successful in combination with nicotine patches (Williams and Foulds 2007). NRT may be more successful at improving abstinence in combination with atypical than with typical antipsychotics (George *et al.* 2000).

Generally, the effects of nicotine from NRT are no different from smoking-derived nicotine. NRT products can cause gastrointestinal disturbance, headache, dizziness, influenza-like symptoms, dry mouth, rash and palpitations. In addition, nasal sprays can cause irritation of nasal mucosa, sneezing, epistaxis and watering eyes. Patches can cause sleep disturbance, nightmares and local skin irritation, and patients with skin disorders should exercise care. Nicotine gum can cause stomach irritation; inhalators can cause coughing; lozenges can cause stomach irritation, thirst, sleep disturbance and nightmares; gum, lozenges, sublingual tablets and inhalators can produce hiccups or throat irritation. Therefore, the choice of which delivery mode to use should be guided by what the patient can tolerate.

Antidepressants

Antidepressants may be beneficial in smoking cessation for at least three reasons. First, nicotine withdrawal may produce depressive symptoms or trigger a major depressive episode, which antidepressants may alleviate. Second, nicotine may have an antidepressant effect that sustains a smoking habit. In this case, antidepressants may substitute for this effect. Lastly, some antidepressants may have a specific inhibiting effect on neural pathways or receptors that underlie nicotine addiction.

A Cochrane systematic review of 90 studies showed that the antidepressants bupropion and nortriptyline double smoking cessation rates but other antidepressants, such as selective serotonin reuptake inhibitors, had no association with cessation rates (Hughes *et al.* 2014). Another study found that bupropion can help to reduce smoking in people with schizophrenia and does not worsen clinical symptoms of the disorder (Evins *et al.* 2005). The action of bupropion and nortriptyline appears to be independent of their antidepressant effect. In any event, you should warn the patient about side effects of antidepressants and take steps to manage them.

Another pharmacological intervention is the use of varenicline, a nicotine receptor partial **agonist**. First, it acts as an agonist by stimulating nicotine receptors to maintain moderate levels of dopamine in the reward system and this counteracts withdrawal symptoms. Second, it acts as an antagonist in the reward system, therefore reducing smoking satisfaction. A Cochrane systematic review with a total of 12,223 participants found that, in comparison to pharmacologically unassisted cessation attempts, varenicline increases smoking cessation threefold. More participants stopped smoking successfully with varenicline than with bupropion (Cahill *et al.* 2012).

Non-pharmacological interventions

Meta-analyses show that simple advice from a health promotion worker has a small but significant effect on smoking cessation by patients (Rice and Stead 2008). However, evidence for efficacy is weaker if the advice is given by nurses whose primary work is not to provide brief interventions and counselling for health promotion or smoking cessation. This calls for nurses to have specialist training in smoking cessation counselling, as it is effective. Other meta-analysis suggests that group therapy and telephone support are effective in long-term smoking cessation (Stead *et al.* 2007). Apart from tobacco dependence, people with mental health problems may abuse non-prescription drugs and this has profound health consequences, as we will discuss next.

Drug abuse and dependence

Under various international treaties, there is a prohibition on the use of certain drugs for non-medical purposes. The main drugs in this category include plant-based drugs such as heroin, cocaine and cannabis, synthetic drugs, including amphetamines, and pharmaceutical drugs such as opioids and benzodiazepines. Drug use disorders directly accounted for almost 20 million disability-adjusted life-years. Worldwide, more people are dependent on opioids and amphetamines than other drugs, with men more likely to be dependent on drugs than women. There are many types of drugs that people misuse and each class may require different pharmacological and non-pharmacological approaches. The types we will look at are stimulants and opiates.

Psychostimulants

Case study

Femi is a 33-year-old man who dropped out of university following repeated admission to hospital for psychosis. At the time, the treatment team felt that the psychosis was mainly due to Femi's incessant use of cannabis. Four years ago, Femi started using crack cocaine because he found it cheap and easily available. He particularly enjoyed the intense pleasurable feeling that he derived from this particular

> *drug. A week ago, he was admitted to hospital following deterioration in his mental state and his mother stated that he was spending most of his time looking for drugs. Lately, he has not been able to get any drugs because he cannot find the money to finance his habit. On admission to hospital, Femi has stated that he feels irritable and depressed.*

Psychostimulants are a group of drugs that people become dependent on or addicted to, as in Femi's case. They excite the central nervous system and produce feelings of alertness and well-being. There are many naturally occurring psychostimulants, including caffeine, nicotine, ephedrine, amphetamine and cocaine.

Cocaine and amphetamines are the two major psychostimulants that people use globally for recreational purposes. Approximately 34 million people used amphetamines and 17 million people used cocaine in 2012 alone. Amphetamines are the second most commonly used illicit drug type worldwide, after cannabis (Degenhardt *et al.* 2014a). Methamphetamine and amphetamine are the most common types of drugs people use and they come in pill, powder or crystalline forms that vary in purity (Degenhardt *et al.* 2014a). Cocaine is a water-soluble white powder with a short half-life and people take cocaine by snorting or injecting. Like most stimulants, it increases levels of dopamine in the reward system in addition to increasing levels of serotonin and noradrenaline. Repeated use of the drug at increasingly high doses leads to a state of increasing irritability, restlessness and paranoia and this may develop into a full-blown paranoid psychosis.

An amalgam reaction of cocaine and baking soda (sodium bicarbonate) produces crack cocaine, a hard brittle crystalline substance. Crack cocaine's absorption into the blood stream is faster than that of cocaine, making it a highly addictive stimulant. Initially, it causes a release of a large amount of dopamine in the reward system, inducing feelings of euphoria, supreme confidence, paranoia, insomnia, alertness, increased energy and loss of appetite. The euphoria usually lasts for up to 10 minutes before dopamine levels in the reward system of the brain plummet, leaving the user feeling low, depressed and craving more crack cocaine. This may partly explain why Femi was feeling depressed and irritable upon admission to hospital. Like most stimulants, crack cocaine causes physical health disorders that include constricted blood vessels, dilated pupils, increased temperature, rapid heart rate and high blood pressure (Figure 7.4). The increase in heart rate and blood pressure can lead to long-term cardiovascular problems.

Another psychostimulant that people commonly use is cannabis and we will look at this next.

Cannabis use

Cannabis is a generic term for marijuana, hashish and hash oil from the *Cannabis sativa* plant. Its use is widespread in all countries. Cannabis dependence accounted for 0.12% of global disability-adjusted life-years in 2010 (Kerridge *et al.* 2014). Regular cannabis use is a clear risk factor for schizophrenia, as current evidence from several systematic reviews suggests (Ben and Potvin 2007; Minozzi *et al.* 2010). Males are twice as likely as females to develop cannabis-related schizophrenia.

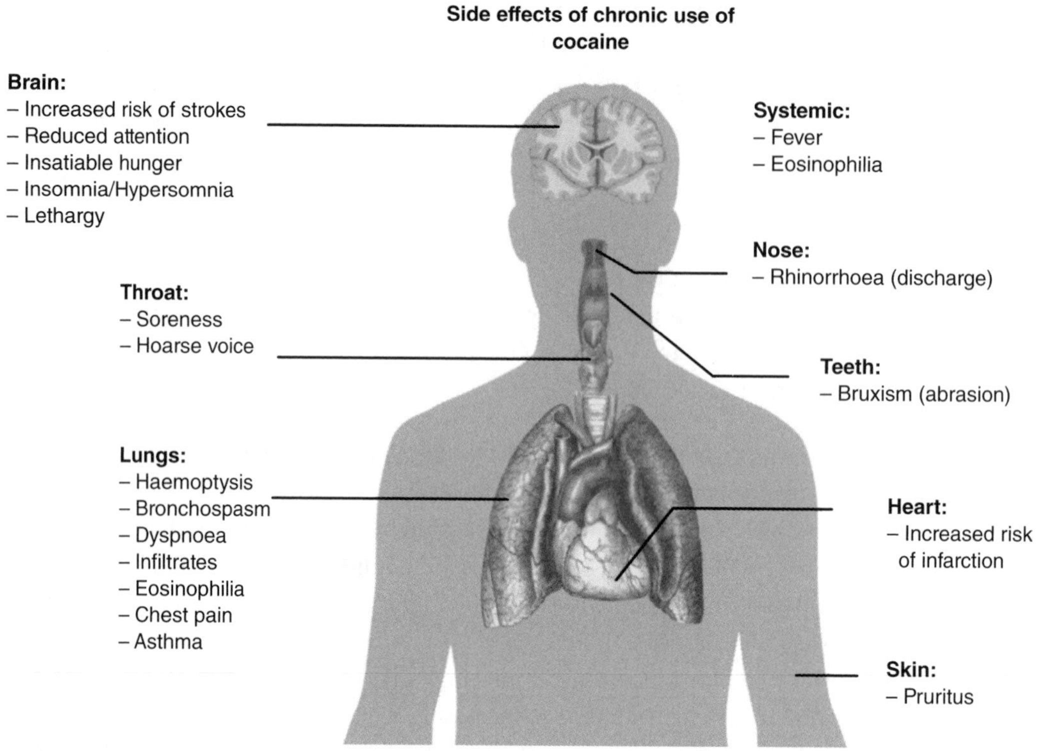

Side effects of chronic use of cocaine

Brain:
– Increased risk of strokes
– Reduced attention
– Insatiable hunger
– Insomnia/Hypersomnia
– Lethargy

Systemic:
– Fever
– Eosinophilia

Nose:
– Rhinorrhoea (discharge)

Throat:
– Soreness
– Hoarse voice

Teeth:
– Bruxism (abrasion)

Lungs:
– Haemoptysis
– Bronchospasm
– Dyspnoea
– Infiltrates
– Eosinophilia
– Chest pain
– Asthma

Heart:
– Increased risk
  of infarction

Skin:
– Pruritus

Figure 7.4: Physical problems resulting from the use of cocaine. (Reproduced from: Häggström M (2014) Medical gallery of Mikael Häggström 2014. Wikiversity Journal of Medicine)

Cannabis produces as many as 60 chemicals (cannabinoids), but we know little about most of them. The most common and powerful cannabinoids are delta-9-tetrahydrocannabinol (THC), cannabidiol and cannabinol. These cannabinoids are able to bind to specific cannabis receptors (endocannabinoid receptors) all over the body and this is the basis of the psychoactive properties of cannabis. The rest of the cannabinoids are either inactive or only weakly active, although they may interact with THC. THC has mild to moderate pain-killing properties and it has other effects that include relaxation, alteration of visual, auditory and olfactory senses, fatigue, and appetite stimulation. It also has clear antiemetic properties.

Cannabis smoke contains thousands of organic and inorganic chemical compounds. The tar in cannabis smoke is similar to tobacco smoke in cigarettes or cigars. Cannabis contains over 50 known carcinogens and these include nitrosamines, reactive aldehydes and polycyclic hydrocarbons, including benzapyrene. Directly inhaled cannabis smoke contains five times as much hydrogen cyanide and 20 times as much ammonia as tobacco smoke. Cannabis has an association with a vast array of physical conditions (Figure 7.5).

Withdrawal from psychostimulants

Stimulant drugs such as amphetamines, cocaine and ecstasy do not produce a major physiological withdrawal syndrome and it is possible to stop them abruptly, as we saw with Femi. However,

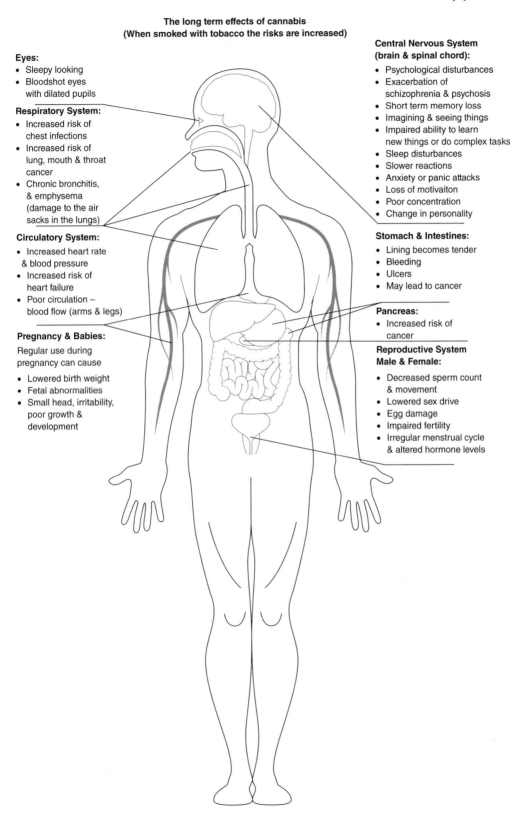

**The long term effects of cannabis
(When smoked with tobacco the risks are increased)**

Eyes:
- Sleepy looking
- Bloodshot eyes with dilated pupils

Respiratory System:
- Increased risk of chest infections
- Increased risk of lung, mouth & throat cancer
- Chronic bronchitis, & emphysema (damage to the air sacks in the lungs)

Circulatory System:
- Increased heart rate & blood pressure
- Increased risk of heart failure
- Poor circulation – blood flow (arms & legs)

Pregnancy & Babies:
Regular use during pregnancy can cause
- Lowered birth weight
- Fetal abnormalities
- Small head, irritability, poor growth & development

Central Nervous System (brain & spinal chord):
- Psychological disturbances
- Exacerbation of schizophrenia & psychosis
- Short term memory loss
- Imagining & seeing things
- Impaired ability to learn new things or do complex tasks
- Sleep disturbances
- Slower reactions
- Anxiety or panic attacks
- Loss of motivaiton
- Poor concentration
- Change in personality

Stomach & Intestines:
- Lining becomes tender
- Bleeding
- Ulcers
- May lead to cancer

Pancreas:
- Increased risk of cancer

Reproductive System Male & Female:
- Decreased sperm count & movement
- Lowered sex drive
- Egg damage
- Impaired fertility
- Irregular menstrual cycle & altered hormone levels

Figure 7.5: The physical and mental health effect of cannabis

people who have regularly used stimulant drugs may experience insomnia and depressed mood when they stop taking the drug. Care and management involve calming and reassuring the patient until the effects wear off. Occasionally, the patient may require oral diazepam (10–20 mg) to help to keep calm, and in severe cases where symptoms persist, the doctor may prescribe an antipsychotic medication.

Where a patient is experiencing low mood, antidepressant medicines can be useful, but many stimulant users just need advice regarding the likely symptoms, and reassurance that they will pass. In Femi's case, you should assess the severity of his depression and look out for suicidal ideation. Occasionally, patients may become acutely suicidal and will require close observation. There is no recognised role for substitute prescribing in the management of stimulant withdrawal.

Rarely, cocaine overdose can result in cardiovascular complications, including arrhythmia, hypertension and cardiac ischaemia. Seizures and hyperpyrexia can also occur. In such cases, treatment is supportive, as there are no specific drugs we use to reverse the effects of cocaine. Some people experience severe distress during or after use of hallucinogenic drugs and may need symptomatic treatment (such as a brief course of a benzodiazepine to reduce anxiety) as well as a safe place to be while the experience passes. THC, the main psychoactive constituent in the cannabis plant, has an extremely low toxicity and poses no threat of death. An early review concluded that no deaths directly due to acute cannabis use have ever been reported (Ashton 2001).

We now turn our attention to opioids.

Opiate abuse and dependence

In 2010, there were 15.5 million opiate-dependent people globally. Regions with the highest opioid dependence are North America, Eastern Europe and Australasia. Opiate dependence is a substantial contributor to the global disease burden; its contribution to premature mortality varies geographically, with North America, Eastern Europe and southern sub-Saharan Africa most strongly affected (Degenhardt *et al.* 2014b).

Opiates are naturally occurring **alkaloids** found in the opium poppy plant. The plant has at least 24 alkaloids but only morphine, codeine and thebaine are psychoactive.

Opiates act as neurotransmitters in neurons that arise from the ventral tegmental area to the nucleus accumbens in the brain. The body produces its own natural opiates such as endorphins or enkephalins that act on a variety of opiate receptors, including the mu (μ), delta (δ) and kappa (κ) receptors. Opiate drugs of abuse like heroin also act in a similar manner by mimicking the body's natural opiates (endorphins or enkephalins), particularly at μ receptors. They induce a very intense but brief euphoria we sometimes call a 'rush' and a profound sense of tranquillity follows which may last several hours. Drowsiness, mood swings, mental clouding, apathy and slowed motor movements can then follow the feeling of tranquillity. In overdose, opiates act as respiratory depressants and can induce coma. Opiates easily cause tolerance and dependence.

Quantitative and systematic review of chronic opioid use suggests that use of these drugs has an association with deficits across a range of different neuropsychological domains. In particular,

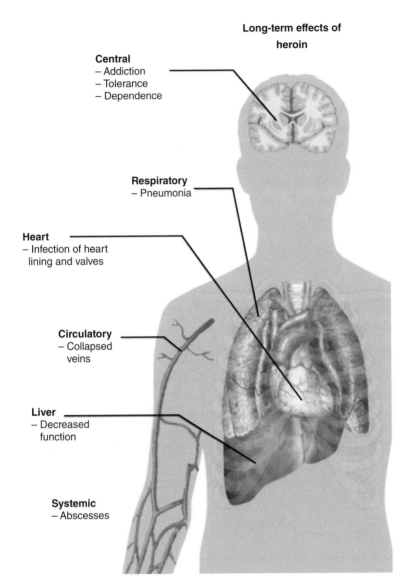

Long-term effects of heroin

Central
– Addiction
– Tolerance
– Dependence

Respiratory
– Pneumonia

Heart
– Infection of heart
lining and valves

Circulatory
– Collapsed
veins

Liver
– Decreased
function

Systemic
– Abscesses

Figure 7.6: The long-term harmful effects of heroin use. (Reproduced from: Häggström M (2014) Medical gallery of Mikael Häggström 2014. Wikiversity Journal of Medicine.)

chronic opiate use has a robust relationship with cognitive impulsivity (risk taking), cognitive flexibility (verbal fluency) and verbal working memory (Baldacchino *et al.* 2012). Other long-term effects of opiates such as heroin are shown in Figure 7.6.

Opiate withdrawal

As with alcohol, one of the first obstacles you may face as a nurse is how to assess opiate withdrawal symptoms. There are clear advantages in using a rating instrument that provides accurate and clinically relevant measurements of opiate withdrawal symptoms. One such instrument is the shortened version of the Opiate Withdrawal Scale (Gossop 1990). This scale (Table 7.2) provides a satisfactory and valid measure of the distress individuals experience when withdrawing from opiates. The scale is straightforward, clinically useful and easy to use and takes less than a minute to complete.

The most commonly selected opioid for detoxification is methadone because it is effective and has good absorption after oral administration. It has a relatively long half-life, therefore once- or twice-daily doses give an extended duration of cover against the more extreme aspects of the withdrawal syndrome (Stahl 2008). To confirm the use of opiates, you will need collaborative evidence in the form of a positive urine test. In addition, you need to observe for positive signs and symptoms of withdrawal and recent sites of injections (depending on the route). The most common symptoms of withdrawal include nausea, stomach cramps, insomnia, muscular tension, muscle spasm/twitching, and aches and pains. Table 7.2 shows the ten items of the Opioid Withdrawal Scale.

Opioid withdrawal reactions are very uncomfortable but are not life-threatening and it is important to ask patients when they had their last dose, as withdrawal symptoms tend to peak at around 32–72 hours after the last dose of opiates was taken. In general, withdrawal symptoms tend to subside after 5 days.

As with anyone suffering from a mental health disorder, the issue of importance in treating opioid withdrawal symptoms is not so much treating the disease state as treating the individual. You should take account of the individual's emotional and spiritual condition as these play an important part in a person's recovery process. During the process of obtaining informed consent from the patient, you should provide detailed information about the detoxification procedure and any possible risks posed. You should also explain about the physical and psychological aspects of opioid withdrawal. Explain the duration of symptoms, their intensity and how to manage these

Symptom	None	Mild	Moderate	Severe
Feeling sick				
Stomach cramps				
Muscle spasms/twitching				
Feeling of coldness				
Heart pounding				
Muscular tension				
Aches and pains				
Yawning				
Runny eyes				
Insomnia/problems sleeping				

Table 7.2: The shortened Opioid Withdrawal Scale

symptoms. It is important that you explain to the patient that there will be loss of tolerance to opioids following detoxification. There is also an increased risk of overdose and death from illicit drug use due to alcohol or benzodiazepine potentiation. You should emphasise the importance of continued support as well as psychosocial and appropriate pharmacological interventions, to maintain abstinence, treat comorbid mental health problems and reduce the risk of adverse outcomes (including death).

Traditionally, we manage the withdrawal from opiates by administering reducing doses of either the opiate of dependence (for example, diamorphine) or, alternatively, an opioid such as methadone. The NICE (2007b) guidelines recommend that methadone or buprenorphine should be the first-line treatment in opioid detoxification. When deciding between these medications, the issues are, first, whether the service user is receiving maintenance treatment with methadone or buprenorphine; if so, opioid detoxification should normally be started with the same medication, and second, the preference of the service user. The prescriber and the patient agree on the choice of opioid for withdrawal state. You should offer advice on aspects of lifestyle that require particular attention during opioid detoxification; these include a balanced diet, adequate hydration, sleep, hygiene and regular physical exercise (see Chapter 9). You should develop a care plan in agreement with the patient to establish and sustain a respectful and supportive relationship to help the patient identify situations or states when he or she is vulnerable to drug misuse and to explore alternative coping strategies, including the involvement of family and carers, so long as confidentiality is maintained.

An important part of recovery from opiates is engagement with self-help groups; you should provide the patient with information about self-help groups such as Narcotics Anonymous.

Before you proceed further, try the activity below.

Activity 7.3 Critical thinking

Ben is a 31-year-old man who has been using illicit drugs since he dropped out of university 11 years ago. He uses a variety of street drugs, including heroin. He informs you that he has been taking methadone as well as illicit drugs until 24 hours before he was admitted to hospital for depression. What should your admission assessment include?

Methadone is a typical example of replacement therapy. Replacement therapy is the use of substances that are similar to, but less addictive than, the drug of abuse. It is the most effective medicine we currently use in detoxification (Faggiano *et al.* 2003). It is a synthetic opiate whose action is very similar to that of heroin, except that it has a longer half-life and does not produce the same euphoric effects as heroin (Mutsatsa, 2011).

As with alcohol, the initial stages of opiate treatment start with the detoxification stage. It is best to carry out this stage in a controlled environment, as evidence suggests that the setting in which we provide treatment has a profound effect, as we see greater adherence and completion rates of detoxification in specialist inpatient services in comparison to general psychiatric ward settings (Strang *et al.* 1997).

The starting dose of methadone is around 10–30 mg daily. In clinical practice, it is important to increase doses slowly under close supervision. It is common for people on methadone therapy to supplement their treatment with other illegal drugs and therefore you should conduct frequent urine analysis to check if the patient is using illegal drugs. We can reduce the doses of methadone gradually over a period of 10–28 days.

You should monitor closely the effects of methadone during the first 2 hours after ingestion because the slow metabolisation of methadone may cause accumulation of the drug in the body and this can cause toxicity. In addition, other drugs may interact with methadone and cause effects on sedation and respiratory depression.

There may be an increased mortality risk during the first weeks of treatment. Meta-analyses conclude that flexible, high-dose strategies are most effective (Bao *et al.* 2009). The recommended dose range is 60–100 mg, sometimes up to 120 mg daily after 7 days of titration. Therapeutic effects of methadone have been reviewed extensively, and two recent systematic Cochrane reviews supported the effectiveness of methadone in terms of an increase in retention in treatment and reduction in heroin use (Faggiano *et al.* 2003; Mattick *et al.* 2009).

Buprenorphine is a synthetic partial agonist that binds to the μ-opioid receptor. Because it is a partial agonist, its maximum effect is less than the maximum effect of full agonists like methadone. It binds to the opioid receptor almost irreversibly and the dissociation from the receptor is slow, giving it a relatively longer half-life. Buprenorphine displaces most opioids from the receptor and, if an individual takes buprenorphine first, other opioids like heroin will be unable to displace it, even in high doses. For these reasons, buprenorphine can precipitate withdrawal in users who have taken other opioids first before buprenorphine, but buprenorphine maintenance may protect patients against overdosing with other opioids. The strong binding reduces the need for additional opioid use, but this may also cause problems in reversing the opioid effects with naltrexone or naloxone. Because it is a partial agonist (it partly stimulates the opioid receptors), it alleviates withdrawal and craving (for full details, see Mutsatsa 2011).

Drug-related deaths from heroin usually involve other drugs too. If you suspect an opioid overdose, you should try to rouse the patient and if you are unsuccessful, then you should call for an ambulance immediately. You should establish a clear airway, adequate ventilation or oxygen therapy if consciousness is impaired. Give naloxone intravenously 0.4–2 mg if the patient is in a coma or respiratory depression is present. Give intramuscularly if no vein is available. Repeat the dose if there is no response within 2 minutes and the patient may need large doses of naloxone (4 mg) if there is severe poisoning. If the patient fails to respond to large doses of naloxone, this may suggest that another central nervous system depressant, or brain damage, is present. You need to stay with the patient until help arrives.

Nursing people with drug misuse problems

- When nursing people with substance misuse-related problems, always ensure that you assess the patient's level of motivation and offer brief interventions focused on motivation to change behaviour.

- It is important that before treatment commencement, you should come to an agreement in the way of an enforceable contract with the patient about the terms and conditions of treatment for withdrawal from substances.

- You should never commence treatment before you do a thorough assessment on the level of substance misuse, symptoms the patient experiences and how frequently, coexistence of mental health problems, family and social support. If a patient who is withdrawing from opioids reports current use of maintenance medication, you should confirm this with the treating doctor or dispensing pharmacy. Confirmation is usually in the form of a faxed letter or prescription.

- Always confirm the use of drugs from a patient by performing a urine drug test to ascertain the main drug of abuse as well as other drugs that the patient may not have reported.

- It is inadvisable to give methadone to a patient taking respiratory depressants such as alcohol or benzodiazepines because the risk of overdose is greatly increased.

- If a patient reports liver function problems, you should withhold giving methadone and report this to the doctor. Renal or hepatic dysfunction interferes with the breakdown of methadone and can result in accumulation of methadone in the plasma, and this can cause an overdose.

- You should be aware that medications used in detoxification are open to misuse and diversion and therefore you need to be vigilant during supervised consumption to limit the risk of concealment.

- For patients on methadone, you should ensure electrocardiogram (ECG) recordings at regular intervals. Some authorities recommend ECGs should be taken prior to methadone commencement and then again after 4 weeks (period of stabilisation) and then at 6–12 months thereafter (Taylor et al., 2007).

Chapter summary

The non-medical use of drugs is a growing problem worldwide and has profound health implications. In people with mental health problems, the misuse of substances is higher in comparison with the general population. Common substances of misuse are alcohol, tobacco, stimulants and opiates. These substances work by increasing dopamine in the mesolimbic reward system and a drop in dopamine in this system leads to withdrawal symptoms. The use of alcohol is widespread: chronic abuse of this substance leads to several physical disorders, including cirrhosis, cancer and gastric problems, and alcohol detoxification includes the use of benzodiazepines. Tobacco use is also widespread but its use can cause many physical diseases, including lung diseases, cancers and circulatory problems. NRT and antidepressants are some of the more effective treatments for tobacco smoking cessation. Opiate misuse presents with many health problems and their use is widespread. The use of methadone for opiate withdrawal is the treatment of choice. Last, though psychostimulants are widely used, there is no known pharmacological intervention for psychostimulant withdrawal.

Activities: brief outline answers

Activity 7.1

The consequences include poor medication adherence, poor physical and mental health, poor self-care, increased suicide risk or aggression, increased sexual behaviour and possible criminal activities.

Activity 7.2

Get a full history of drinking and the reason for drinking. How was the habit financed, as this may lead to further revelations of financial difficulties; elicit symptoms using a scale, discuss detoxification options and inform doctor. Most importantly, provide support and reassurance and make a full documentation.

Activity 7.3

You need to assess for symptoms of withdrawal, possibly using a rating scale. You need to take a history of drug usage that includes the type of drug, the quantity taken a day and approximately how much money the patient spent a day on drugs. Take a history of methadone taking, the name and address of the prescribing doctor, the name and address of the dispensing pharmacy and it is vitally important to confirm the prescription or dispensing record, usually by way of fax. Lastly you need to confirm which drugs the patient has been taking using a drug urine analysis.

Further reading

Mutsatsa S (2011) *Medicines Management in Mental Health Nursing: Transforming practice.* Exeter: Learning Matters.

A book on medication management aimed at student nurses that is easy to understand and apply.

Useful websites

http://www.mentalhealth.org.uk/help-information/mental-health-a-z/D/drugs

This website provides help, advice and information for those suffering from mental health problems, including substance abuse.

http://www.drugabuse.gov/publications/drugfacts/comorbidity-addiction-other-mental-disorders

This website provides very useful information on substance misuse.

http://www.drugabuse.gov

This website gives information on drug abuse in an easy-to-understand way.

http://www.nice.org.uk/PHI004

This NICE website gives information on different interventions for people who misuse substances.

Chapter 8
Side effects of psychotropic drugs and their management

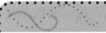

NMC Standards for Pre-registration Nursing Education

This chapter will address the following competencies:

Domain 1: Professional values

Generic standard for competence
All nurses must act first and foremost to care for and safeguard the public. They must practise autonomously and be responsible and accountable for safe, compassionate, person-centred, evidence-based nursing that respects and maintains dignity and human rights. They must show professionalism, integrity, and work within recognised professional, ethical and legal frameworks. They must work in partnership with other health and social care professionals and agencies, service users, their carers and families in all settings, including the community, ensuring that decisions about care are shared.

NMC Essential Skills Clusters

This chapter will address the following ESCs:

1. As partners in the care process, people can trust a newly registered graduate nurse to provide collaborative care based on the highest standards, knowledge and competence.
9. People can trust the newly registered graduate nurse to treat them as partners and work with them to make a holistic and systematic assessment of their needs; to develop a personalised plan that is based on mutual understanding and respect for their individual situation promoting health and well-being, minimising risk of harm and promoting their safety at all times.

Chapter aims

By the end of the chapter, you should be able to:

* describe the different types of psychotropic medication and their mechanism of action;
* understand psychotropic drug side effects both routine and in emergency;
* advise patients on how to manage psychotropic side effects.

Introduction

> ### Case study
>
> *Jude is a 26-year-old male who recently moved back in with his parents after his fiancée was killed in a road accident 6 months ago. Since the accident, Jude has been plagued with nightmares about the accident almost every night. He had to leave his job because the accident scene was very close to where he worked and he has since avoided that entire area of town. Normally an outgoing, fun-loving person, Jude became increasingly withdrawn, 'jumpy' and irritable since his fiancée's death. He stopped going to the gym, playing rugby or playing his guitar. He was referred to the mental health outpatient clinic where he was diagnosed with posttraumatic stress disorder (PTSD) and was prescribed olanzapine 10 mg, which he takes at night. He has noticed some improvement in his mental state. However, he has recently been complaining of troubling side effects, including weight gain, drowsiness, dry mouth and constipation.*

It is difficult to imagine practising modern mental health nursing without relying on psychotropic medication, whose effects have revolutionised the theory and practice of mental health nursing. Psychotropic medication has been available for over five decades, and despite ubiquitous use, there are problems with safe and effective application, as in Jude's case. Psychotropic medications, like any other medication, have side effects and Jude's case demonstrates this point. The majority of the side effects are mild, transient and tolerable. However, some are profound and can even be fatal as they can affect neurotransmitter systems; their effects extend beyond the brain to other systems and organs in the body. In the case of Jude, the primary aim of the olanzapine was to treat PTSD, but this medication had additional effects, including on Jude's autonomous nervous system, giving rise to constipation and other problems.

The management of side effects of psychotropic medication is therefore an important part of the treatment plan and this is the area we will explore in this chapter. The plan should include the evaluation of side effects, and this is frequently a part of the quality-of-life assessment. This is because the frequency and severity of side effects may play a role in the effectiveness and cost analysis of the treatment with a particular psychotropic medication. Jude is unlikely to enjoy the full benefit of medication treatment if he is feeling drowsy and constipated for a significant portion of the day. This makes the correct diagnosis and assessment of side effects an essential part of quality-of-life enhancement. However, many side effects and symptoms of psychotropic medication are similar to symptoms of mental health disorders and this poses specific problems.

The overlapping nature of pathology and treatment side effects

One of the greatest challenges in the treatment of mental health disorders is discriminating between symptoms intrinsic to a person's illness and potential treatment side effects. For example, treatment with antipsychotic medication can induce akathisia, but akathisia is difficult to distinguish from psychotic agitation, anxiety or manic symptoms. In the case of depression, symptoms like lethargy and lack of sleep that are typical of bipolar depression can easily be mistaken for antidepressant side effects. Similarly, if symptoms worsen after commencement of treatment, it may be difficult to differentiate whether this reflects an adverse medication side effect or simply a worsening of the symptoms. For example, a depressed patient may present with agitation, insomnia and suicidal ideation after a period of treatment. In any event, a patient who is complaining of side effects is communicating important information about himself/herself which you must take seriously.

In clinical practice, some patients complain of medication side effects that are not consistent with the drug's pharmacological profile. For example, it has been known for some time that some patients report side effects from placebos (nocebo effect) and this elicits a unique type of concern that individuals might have for their physical health. By definition, physical complaints from placebos are not pharmacodynamic in origin, yet if a person can attribute these to treatment, it can provide validation and legitimacy to the individual's subjective sense of suffering.

Scenario

Imagine you are nursing Fred, 67, who reports side effects which are frankly implausible considering the drug treatment he is on. Should you challenge the validity of this dubious self-reporting? You decide to assure Fred that the condition poses no serious medical hazard. Fred later complains of distress arising from the adverse effect, and you decide to advocate for an alternative treatment because if Fred continues with the existing therapy, he may have a negative therapeutic experience.

Negative therapeutic reaction and experience

From a psychodynamic perspective, a negative therapeutic experience occurs when a patient develops an incongruous worsening of symptoms in response to accurate treatment interventions. Any treatment regimen can result in adverse side effects at any time and, as a nurse, you will at times see patients whose symptoms clearly worsen in response to a medication that aims to ameliorate their condition. An intensification of depression, low mood and feelings of guilt during antidepressant therapy is a useful example. It is therefore tempting to think this is due to lack of medication efficacy but a psychodynamic perspective is equally valid. Freud, as cited by Levy (1982), describes the above phenomenon as *an unconscious expression of guilt or masochism on the part of the patient whose symptoms worsen because the prospect of improvement is contrary to an unconscious investment in the person's own suffering.*

You can imagine that Fred might describe a seemingly endless stream of physical ailments that he links to treatment, all the while developing a parallel sense of frustration, resentment and loss of sympathy from the healthcare team. This will evidently make the interaction between Fred and the nurses personally and psychodynamically complex. You need to appreciate the psychological context of Fred's presenting symptoms to avoid his treatment becoming a relentless and seemingly fruitless effort to combat side effects or to identify less harmful medicines while the patient is deriving no tangible treatment benefits.

To break this cycle, you should seek consultation or, in certain instances, you may honestly acknowledge to the patient that existing treatments may not be capable of providing tangible benefits that outweigh side effects. In such circumstances, you should discuss alternative therapies with the patient, including psychotherapy, as this may hold greater prospects for success (Goldberg and Ernst 2012).

The general principles of side-effect management

The person who is under treatment has important and clinically relevant characteristics that will have an impact both on the course of the person's illness and the person's treatment behaviour. Put differently, it is important to collaborate with patients so that they can implement the treatment plan. This involves proactive strategies for managing side effects, as they are a major obstacle in adherence with treatment and this affects the optimum benefit to treatment. Furthermore, the education process must be ongoing and you cannot accomplish this in a single encounter or a single hand-out (Frank 1997). We will look at your role in educating patients about their medication later.

Before the commencement of treatment, you may find it helpful to ask the patient to make a list of troublesome symptoms that the medication should target. Second, and perhaps critically, when a patient complains of adverse side effects, it is important for you to establish whether they were present or absent before treatment. If the problem was absent before treatment, it is likely that it is a medication side effect. In the case of illness symptoms that intensify during treatment with medication, this differentiation can be particularly difficult. For example, insomnia that predates the initiation of some antidepressants like selective serotonin reuptake inhibitors (SSRIs), which then worsens after commencement of treatment, may be particularly difficult to attribute to side effects or worsening of mental state.

Thirdly, it is important for you to gather information about the patient's previous medication and past adverse side effects and make a summary of past medications, dates taken, dosages, benefits and side effects. This information will help you understand previous treatment complications or failures, reasons for non-adherence and the patient's ability to tolerate side effects. It will also help you to recognise potential patterns or sensitivities that may heighten the patient's expectations about future potential side effects or concerns. Before you read further, let's look at tolerance of side effects more closely.

Activity 8.1   *Critical thinking*

What factors may influence intolerance to side effects?

There are outline answers to all the activities at the end of the chapter.

You should discuss side effects in a positive way that minimises over-concern. Discuss common side effects and what to do if these occur, but don't read out all the possible side effects that are in the *British National Formulary*. Merely listing the side effects is likely to increase the patient's anxiety. Rather, for those who have sleep problems you could present sedation as a beneficial effect. Alternatively, you could suggest that, if daytime sedation becomes a problem, then the patient should let the treating staff know with a view to reviewing the medication. For some patients, however, medication dose reduction or tapering off is not a clinically viable option, given the seriousness of some mental health problems and the high risk of relapse and significant harm to self or to others. Where anticholinergic side effects such as blurred vision and dry mouth are concerned, you could describe these as usually bothersome and you can advise patients that these effects are usually worse during the first 2 weeks of treatment, with some tolerance developing if they stay on the same dosage. Overall, there are different ways to educate a patient about side effects but the key part of the process is the discussion of the risks and benefits that treatment poses and obtaining informed consent. Always document your discussion with a patient regarding side effects and consent issues.

You should be alert to the presence of pharmacodynamic inconsistencies when a patient is complaining about adverse side effects, such as co-occurring problems that have opposing mechanisms of action. For example, the co-occurrence of dry mouth with diarrhoea or excessive salivation with constipation should alert you that you need to probe patients further to elicit other underlying problems they may have. In this case, you should validate the patient's experience rather than say that it is impossible, as the medicine has no cholinergic effects. In the assessment of side effects, a good starting point is to ascertain if the side effects bear any relationship to treatment. The best approach is to use a method devised by Naranjo *et al.* (1981). The Naranjo Adverse Drug Reactions Probability Scale (Table 8.1) is a simple and widely used non-specific scale.

	Question	Yes	No	Do not know	Score
1	Are there previous *conclusive* reports on this reaction?	+1	0	0	
2	Did the adverse event occur after the suspected drug was administered?	+2	−1	0	
3	Did the adverse reaction improve when the drug was discontinued or a *specific* antagonist was administered?	+1	0	0	
4	Did the adverse reaction reappear when the drug was readministered?	+2	−1	0	
5	Are there alternative causes (other than the drug) that could have on their own caused the reaction?	−1	+2	0	
6	Did the reaction reappear when a placebo was given?	−1	+1	0	

(Continued)

(Continued)

	Question	Yes	No	Do not know	Score
7	Was the drug detected in the blood (or other fluids) in concentrations known to be toxic?	+1	0	0	
8	Was the reaction more severe when the dose was increased or less severe when the dose was decreased?	+1	0	0	
9	Did the patient have a similar reaction to the same or similar drugs in *any* previous exposure?	+1	0	0	
10	Was the adverse event confirmed by any objective evidence?	+1	0	0	
	Total score				

Scoring

9 or more = definite adverse drug reaction; 5–8 = probable adverse drug reaction; 1–4 = possible adverse drug reaction; 0 = doubtful adverse drug reaction.

Table 8.1: The Naranjo Adverse Drug Reactions Probability Scale (reproduced from Naranjo et al. 1981)

In addition to the use of this scale to assist with adverse side-effect management, you may find the 'ten commandments' of wise drug management helpful in minimising adverse side effects (Keshavan 1992):

1. Know your patient well.
2. Work on offering a treatment package, not just a prescription.
3. Educate the patient.
4. Assist the patient in choosing the right medicine.
5. Ensure that the patient takes the medicines correctly.
6. In collaboration with the prescriber, ensure the patient is on as few drugs as possible.
7. Assist in ensuring that treatment is tailored to the patient's needs.
8. Have a good knowledge of the medicine the patient is taking.
9. Be vigilant of side effects.
10. Always consider the patient's viewpoint, as it is critical.

We can now turn to specific side effects of psychotropic medications and their management and we will start with extrapyramidal side effects (EPSEs).

Extrapyramidal side effects and their management

EPSEs are various movement disorders that are caused by the antagonistic action of psychotropic medication on the extrapyramidal system or the nigrostriatal dopamine pathway. Commonly used psychotropic medicines have an association with EPSE. Other dopamine antagonists that cause EPSEs are metoclopramide and most types of antidepressants, including SSRIs, tricyclic and tetracyclic antidepressants. The most common cause of EPSEs is antipsychotic medication. Positron emission tomography studies suggest that, when antipsychotics block more than 80% of striatal dopamine receptors, EPSEs develop (Kapur and Remington 2001). At clinically effective doses, some of the newer atypical antipsychotic medicines block less than 80% of dopamine receptors, which may partly explain their clinical efficacy with minimal EPSEs.

EPSE can take several forms, including dystonia, akathisia, parkinsonism and tardive dyskinesia. We will look at these problems now in turn.

Dystonia

The key features of dystonia are involuntary contractions or spasms of the muscles affecting the head, spine and extremities, and the facial, laryngeal and neck muscles, which can be painful and frightening. For example, the jaw may open involuntarily, which can result in dislocation. Laryngeal spasms can result in difficulties in swallowing and this can be life-threatening. About 10% of all patients experience dystonia as an adverse effect of conventional antipsychotics, although all classes of antipsychotics cause dystonia. Acute dystonic reactions typically occur within hours of initiating treatment, particularly with intramuscular injections of high-potency antipsychotics. Young men below the age of 40 years are most at risk. An oculogyric crisis is a type of dystonic reaction that involves a sustained involuntary upward deviation of the eyes and all classes of antipsychotics cause the condition. Other types of medication, like SSRI, lithium and carbamazepine, can cause oculogyric crisis. Although the diagnosis of acute dystonia is relatively straightforward, there are situations when the condition has been mistaken for hysterical reactions, tetanus or even meningitis.

In the event of an acute dystonic reaction occurring, you should reassure the patient and take necessary steps to alleviate the condition. Dystonic reactions generally respond dramatically well to anticholinergic medication, such as intramuscular injection of procyclidine, and this is the treatment of choice (Hansen *et al.* 1997). Most patients respond within 5 minutes and are symptom-free by 15 minutes. If there is no response the dose can be repeated after 10 minutes, but if that does not work then the diagnosis is probably wrong. Before you read further, you need to think more about the route of administration.

Activity 8.2   *Critical thinking*

We treat a severe dystonic reaction with an intramuscular dose of an anticholinergic medication. Why is it not advisable to give an oral tablet of an anticholinergic in severe dystonia?

Some patients can respond well to benzodiazepines, diphenhydramine or biperiden. Apart from assisting with giving medication to ameliorate the condition, your role during acute dystonia is to provide as much reassurance as possible. Many patients rightly find the condition frightening and you should emphasise that it is temporary and will improve after treatment. However, in some patients, persistent dystonia (tardive dystonia) may occur due to chronic exposure to anti-psychotics. If what appears to be chronic dystonia does not respond to standard treatment, the condition might not be due to antipsychotics and such illnesses might include Wilson's disease, Huntington's disease or idiopathic torsion dystonia.

Another troublesome EPSE is akathisia, which we will look at next.

Akathisia

The term akathisia derives from the Greek and means 'not to sit still'. It is a subjective feeling of muscular discomfort and inner restlessness: a compulsion to move the legs when sitting and inability to stand still in one place are the most common features of akathisia (Barnes and Braude 1985). Theodore Van Putten was the first to identify subtle subjective akathisia as a behaviourally toxic component of psychosis treatment (Sachdev 1995). It is probably the most disabling and intolerable side effect that develops early during treatment with psychotropic medication.

Akathisia often develops in patients taking all types of antipsychotics or during rapid dose esca-lation. Second-generation antipsychotics like risperidone, ziprasidone and aripiprazole possess a higher risk than olanzapine, whereas quetiapine and clozapine present the lowest risk (Poyurovsky 2010) (Table 8.2). About 25% of patients on first-generation antipsychotic treat-ment will develop akathisia (Halstead *et al.* 1994). Women are twice as likely as men to experience akathisia. Affective disorder patients on second-generation antipsychotics are more vulnerable to developing akathisia in comparison with patients suffering from schizophrenia (Gao *et al.* 2008). To a lesser extent, akathisia can develop with all types of antidepressants.

Akathisia often resembles psychotic agitation and there is an association between higher doses of antipsychotic medication and the condition. It often exists in tandem with other EPSEs, like par-kinsonism, dystonia and tardive dykinesia. The pathophysiology of akathisia is not clear but one theory suggests it may involve an imbalance of several neurotransmitters, including dopamine, acetylcholine, gamma-aminobutyric acid (GABA), noradrenaline, serotonin and neuropeptides.

First-generation antipsychotics	Second-generation antipsychotics
Chlorpromazine	Clozapine
Thioridazine	Olanzapine
Trifluperazine	Quetiapine
Fluphenazine	Risperidone
Haloperidol	Amisulpiride
Clopixol	Asenapine
Depixol	Iloperidone
Sulpiride	Paliperidone

Table 8.2: Classification of antipsychotic drugs

For example, dopamine antagonism may affect GABA levels in the pallidus or noradrenaline levels in the locus coeruleus. Overall, dopamine blockade is *necessary* in the development of akathisia but not *sufficient* to explain this condition completely.

The essential features of antipsychotic-induced acute akathisia are subjective complaints of restlessness and at least one of the following observed movements:

- fidgety movements or swinging of the legs while seated;
- rocking from foot to foot or 'walking on the spot' while standing;
- pacing to relieve the restlessness, or an inability to sit or stand still for at least several minutes (Sachdev, 1995).

For best results, you should use a rating scale such as the Barnes Akathisia Rating scale (Barnes 1989).

The first line of managing akathisia is the discontinuation of the offending medication. An atypical antipsychotic with a lower propensity to induce akathisia may be a better alternative. In cases where this is not possible, benzodiazepines like diazepam or beta-blockers like propranolol are first-line treatments for akathisia. If the akathisia appears to have its roots in imbalance of the noradrenergic system, then beta-blockers usually work better. Patients who have symptoms of parkinsonism together with akathisia (approximately 65% of patients) may respond to anticholinergic medication like procyclidine (Iqbal *et al.* 2007).

By far the most promising treatment for akathisisa is the use of antidepressants like mirtazapine, trazodone and mianserin that antagonise the serotonin (5-HT$_{2A}$) receptor. A systematic review of six randomised controlled trials found that 5-HT$_{2A}$ antagonists are effective in the treatment of antipsychotic-induced akathisia (Laoutidis and Luckhaus 2014). You are likely to assist in administration of medication and observe for further side effects. Because of the disabling nature of akathisia, you should provide adequate support and reassurance to your patient.

Parkinsonism

Parkinsonism is a complication of antipsychotic treatment as well as of antidepressants, calcium channel antagonists, gastrointestinal prokinetics like domperidone, antiepileptic drugs and many other compounds that interfere with the dopamine system. It occurs in about 15% of patients and it usually develops within 5–90 days of treatment initiation. The risk factors for the development of the condition include older age, female sex, presence of cognitive impairment, the use of high-potency antipsychotics like haloperidol and a genetic predisposition (Lopez-Sendon *et al.* 2012).

The pathophysiology of drug-induced parkinsonism involves a decrease in the activity of the nigrostriatal dopamine pathway due to the action of these medicines. This decrease in activity causes a compensatory increase in the acetylcholine (cholinergic) activity and this may account for some of the symptoms of drug-induced parkinsonism.

The cardinal features of this syndrome include muscle stiffness, cogwheel rigidity, shuffling gait, stooped posture and drooling, mask-like facies, slowness of movements (bradykinesia) and ataraxia (indifference towards the environment). The tremor is more prominent in the distal part of the upper extremities and is present even when the person is resting. Parkinsonism that is due to antipsychotics is often mistaken for the negative-deficit syndrome of schizophrenia or for depression.

The three critical steps in the management of drug-induced parkinsonism include the reduction in the medication dosage, administering anticholinergic medication and changing the antipsychotic medication. The first step is to reduce the dosage of the medicine or administer a concomitant anticholinergic dose of procyclidine trihexyphenidyl, benztropine or amantadine. Because these anticholinergic medications block acetylcholine receptors (antimuscarinic), they cause uncomfortable side effects such as dry mouth, constipation and blurred vision. You should encourage the patient to drink sufficient fluids to counteract these effects. If the symptoms persist and the patient finds them intolerable, you should discuss this with the prescriber with a view to switching to another medication that has a lower propensity for causing these side effects. For example, if a patient develops parkinsonism on risperidone, s/he might switch to less offending medicines such as clozapine or quetiapine. Quetiapine may produce fewer parkinsonian effects than other medicines like paliperidone, aripiprazole and risperidone (Asmal *et al.* 2013).

We now turn our attention to tardive dyskinesia.

Tardive dyskinesia

Case study

Deirdre is a 42-year-old woman with a 16-year history of paranoid schizophrenia. After 10 years of treatment with haloperidol decanoate, a first-generation antipsychotic drug, she developed involuntary movements with tongue chewing, lip puckering, jaw stiffness and finger piano playing.

Haloperidol was gradually reduced and replaced by Risperdal Consta, a depot injection formulation of risperidone. The dyskinetic movements resolved over the following 3 months, and Deirdre remained stable for 4 years.

Tardive dyskinesia is a complex involuntary movement disorder that typically occurs in patients taking psychotropic medication, particularly antipsychotics. Schonecker published the original description of tardive dyskinesia in 1957, about 5 years after the commencement of antipsychotic treatment. Tardive dyskinesia consists of abnormal involuntary, irregular choreoathetoid movements of the muscles of the head, limbs and trunk. Perioral movements are the most common and they include darting, twisting and protruding movements of the tongue, chewing and lateral jaw movements, lip puckering and facial grimacing. Finger movements and hand clenching are also common. We see that Deirdre has most of these symptoms but they are rarely disabling and usually do not bother the patient, although they are of concern to family members. If they are clinically significant, the patient may have problems with swallowing and speech, resulting in speech difficulties and loss of weight.

Tardive dyskinesia has an insidious onset, rarely occurring before 6 months from the onset of treatment with first-generation antipsychotics, as in Deirdre's case. The incidence of tardive dyskinesia is 3–5% for those patients on first-generation antipsychotics but can be as high as 32% after 5 years' exposure to first-generation antipsychotic treatment, as in the case of Deirdre. In the elderly, tardive dyskinesia may develop in as many as 53% of patients after 3 years of cumulative exposure to conventional antipsychotic usage (Woerner *et al.* 1998).

A lower incidence of tardive dyskinesia can occur with second-generation antipsychotics, particularly clozapine, quetiapine or olanzapine. However, virtually all antipsychotics can induce tardive dyskinesia. In particular, those with high potency or tight binding affinity to the dopamine receptor (like haloperidol or risperidone and aripiprazole for the second-generation antipsychotics) have a higher propensity to cause tardive dyskinesia. It subsequently develops into a full syndrome which can persist for years, even after discontinuation of the antipsychotic medication (Kim *et al.* 2014).

The risk factors for tardive dyskinesia are as follows:

- older age;
- female sex;
- African origin;
- prolonged use of antipsychotics;
- pre-existing mood disorder;
- cognitive disturbance;
- alcohol and substance misuse;
- concomitant use of lithium and antiparkinsonian medication;
- diabetes;
- HIV-positive;
- use of high-potency antipsychotics.

Currently, it is not clear why tardive dyskinesia occurs but there are several explanatory models in existence. The most prominent theories include dopamine receptor supersensitivity, GABA depletion, acetylcholine deficiency, neurotoxicity and oxidative stress, changes in synaptic plasticity and defective neuroadaptive signalling. Of these, the dopamine supersensitivity hypothesis is the most promising. This theory proposes that chronic dopamine antagonism (by psychotropics) results in gradual hypersensitization of dopamine receptors; evidence in support of this theory comes from animal studies but direct evidence in humans is at an embryonic stage.

The management of tardive dyskinesia starts with correct assessment of symptoms and you can do this using a rating scale. The Abnormal Involuntary Movement Scale (Guy 1976) is probably the most widely used scale for the assessment to establish the presence of tardive dyskinesia. This 12-item scale records details of the occurrence of dyskinesia in patients: each item is rated on a five-point scale (from 0 = none to 4 = severe).

The treatment of tardive dyskinesia includes gradual reduction of any anticholinergic co-medications as the primary step before switching from the offending medicine to an atypical antipsychotic. Switching from first-generation to second-generation remains the most effective treatment of antipsychotic-induced tardive dyskinesia. Determining which second-generation antipsychotic to use depends on the patient's clinical profile and the specific second-generation medication pharmacological profile. If the switch fails to improve tardive dyskinesia symptoms, it is usual for the prescriber to consider another second-generation medicine. In particular, clozapine has a lower risk of tardive dyskinesia and reduces dyskinetic movements in patients with tardive dyskinesia. A review of 15 randomised controlled trials and 28 case reports concluded that clozapine is useful at reducing tardive syndromes in the dose range of 200–300 mg/day and the beneficial effect is usually shown within 4–12 weeks of initiation (Hazari *et al.* 2013).

Next, there is emerging evidence that tetrabenazine is effective for the treatment of movement disorders, including tardive dyskinesia. A recent review of literature concludes that tetrabenazine is a credible alternative for the treatment of dystonia, tardive dyskinesia and Huntington's chorea (Chen *et al.* 2012). Preliminary results from randomised controlled trials suggest a place in the treatment of tardive dyskinesia for vitamin E, ginkgo biloba, vitamin B_6/branched-chain amino acids, donepezil and melatonin, levetiracetam and amantadine (Rana *et al.* 2013). A point you should remind your patient of is that none of the available pharmacological options for the treatment of tardive dyskinesia reduces symptoms dramatically or halts symptom progression significantly. This condition remains intransigent and there is no reliable or well-proven treatment.

Non-extrapyramidal side effects

Apart from extrapyramidal effects, all types of psychotropic medication can cause a range of other adverse effects that have the potential to inflict discomfort and diminish the quality of life of patients who take them over the long term. Of particular significance are cardiovascular, endocrinological, metabolic, hepatic and haematological side effects. Various psychotropics differ substantially with regard to their tendency to induce these side effects. Potentially the most dangerous side effect is their propensity to induce cardiovascular effects.

Cardiovascular effects

Cardiovascular effects can be a direct result from hypotension and anticholinergic-induced tachycardia (Arana 2000). As previously mentioned, there is current concern and focus over the prevalence of cardiovascular disease in people with mental health problems (see Chapter 1). Although this high prevalence is due to a combination of factors, such as lifestyle and biological factors, we have known for a long time that psychotropic medication and antipsychotics in particular have an association with cardiovascular disorders.

In general, psychotropic medicines that have an affinity for the acetylcholine receptors (antimuscarinic and anticholinergic) can cause cardiovascular complications. These psychotropics include low-potency first-generation antipsychotics, second-generation antipsychotics, tricyclic antidepressants, non-selective monoamine oxidase inhibitors and all antiparkinsonian medicines. Specifically, second-generation antipsychotic medicines like olanzapine, risperidone and quetiepine are a chemically diverse group of medicines that vary in their effect on the cardiovascular system in type and degree. One cardiovascular risk that is common to most antipsychotics is sudden unexpected death.

Reports of sudden unexpected deaths due to antipsychotics began in the early 1960s. There are several mechanisms whereby antipsychotics in particular can cause sudden death. One common mechanism is that antipsychotics cause QT_c elongation, which can lead to *torsade de pointes*. The main feature of *torsade de pointes* is ventricular tachycardia that has distinct characteristics on the electrocardiogram (ECG). The ventricular tarchycardia can develop into ventricular arrhythmia, which ultimately leads to ventricular fibrillation and sudden death. Other cardiovascular effects of antipsychotics, and of second-generation antipsychotics in particular, are deviations in blood pressure and in rare cases, congestive heart failure, myocarditis and sudden death. In addition, all second-generation antipsychotics, with the exception of ziprasidone and aripiprazole, increase serum triglycerides to an extent. Specifically, very high levels of triglycerides (hypertriglyceridaemia) occur predominantly with clozapine and olanzapine.

Risk factors for adverse cardiovascular effects that we associate with the use of second-generation antipsychotic medicines include advanced age, autonomic nervous system dysfunction, pre-existing cardiovascular disease, female gender, electrolyte imbalances (particularly low calcium and magnesium), elevated serum antipsychotic drug concentrations, genetic characteristics and the psychiatric illness itself.

To minimise the cardiovascular effects of antipsychotic medication, you should check the patient's baseline vital signs, electrolytes and ECG prior to commencing medication. Check these regularly and inform the patient about the potential for cardiac problems (see Chapters 4 and 9).

We will now turn our attention to discussing the endocrinological effects of psychotropic medication.

Endocrinological effects

Psychotropic medicines induce a wide range of adverse hormonal (endocrinological) and metabolic effects. Some of these psychotropic medicines include antipsychotics, mood stabilisers and antidepressants. Common metabolic and hormonal effects that these medicines induce include elevated levels of prolactin, calcium, glucose, ketoacidosis and weight gain. These effects are mainly due to the antagonistic effects of psychotropic medication on the tuberoinfundibular dopamine pathway.

The blockade of the tuberoinfundibular pathway by psychotropic medications increases prolactin production (hyperprolactinaemia). Hyperprolactinaemia occurs when prolactin plasma concentration exceeds 20 µg/L, but clinically significant symptoms are unlikely to occur until levels reach 30–60 µg/L (Arana 2000). Hyperprolactinaemia causes irregular or absence of menstruation in women, spontaneous flow of milk from the nipple (galactorrhoea) and impotence in males. As many as 50% of men taking antipsychotics experience impotence and ejaculatory problems due an increase in prolactin. Women may experience orgasmic dysfunction and reduced libido, possibly due to the alpha-adrenergic activity of antipsychotics and calcium channel blockade.

In addition to the antipsychotic action on the tuberoinfundibular pathway, SSRI antidepressants can cause various forms of sexual dysfunction, such as inability to achieve an orgasm, erectile dysfunction and diminished sexual appetite. Recent evidence suggests that such side effects occur in 17–41% of patients taking antidepressants (Landen *et al.* 2005). Antidepressants' side effects are due to their stimulation of postsynaptic 5-HT$_2$ and 5-HT$_3$ receptors by serotonin. The stimulation leads to a decrease in dopamine and noradrenaline release from the substantia nigra and this leads to sexual dysfunction. Sexual side effects can be intolerable to many patients but healthcare professionals often fail to ask about sexual dysfunction and patients tend not to report these types of side effects to their professional carers spontaneously. Before you read further, please take part in the activity below.

Activity 8.3 — *Critical thinking*

Chris, a 26-year-old man who suffers from schizophrenia, has been started on a depot injection of haloperidol decanoate. Recently, he has complained that he 'has no genitals' and 'is turning into a woman'. This is out of his delusional system and the treatment team feels that the current depot dose is not sufficient and therefore the dose should be increased. Do you have any misgivings about this?

High-potency first-generation antipsychotics like haloperidol pose the greatest risk of causing hyperprolactinaemia, although some second-generation antipsychotics, particularly risperidone and paliperidone, increase prolactin secretion. Aripiprazole, clozapine, quetiapine and ziprasidone have little effect on prolactin levels. Typically, antipsychotic-associated hyperprolactinaemia begins within days of treatment initiation and persists throughout treatment. It gradually disappears after discontinuing treatment.

When a patient appears to be suffering from hyperprolactinaemia-related side effects like sexual dysfunction, you should discuss this with the patient as well as the prescriber. A starting point is to test prolactin levels to ascertain if this is above the threshold. You should provide explanations and reassurance to the patient where necessary. If prolactin levels are high, you should discuss this with the patient and prescriber with a view to lowering the medication dose of the offending medication if possible. If this is not possible, then you should discuss and advise the patient that there are other types of medication that have less propensity for causing sexual dysfunction, such as aripiprazole, clozapine, quetiapine or moderate doses of olanzapine. In some instances, it may be possible to prescribe dopamine agonists that suppress prolactin secretion, such as bromocriptine, cabergoline or pergolide. You should however advise the patient that these dopamine agonist medications can increase agitation, psychosis or mania, particularly if the patient does not continue with adequate treatment with an antipsychotic or mood stabiliser.

Weight gain is another important side effect of psychotropic medication and we will turn to this next.

Weight gain

One of the commonest adverse side effects of treatment with medicines that block the dopamine receptor system is weight gain. When chlorpromazine was introduced in the 1950s, most patients gained weight and similar problems have occurred to varying degrees with antidepressants, mood stabilisers and all antipsychotics.

Excessive weight gain renders the patient vulnerable to metabolic illnesses. Such illnesses include cardiovascular diseases and non-insulin-dependent diabetes (see Chapters 4 and 5). A meta-analysis found that second-generation antipsychotics such as olanzapine and clozapine were associated with a higher incidence of inducing diabetes in patients (Newcomer 2005). In spite of the strong evidence suggesting that weight gain and metabolic problems present a serious problem for people on psychotropic medication, screening practices are often incomplete or inconsistent. Most recommended interventions are the provision of dietary advice, physical activity and psychoeducation of the patient and family.

You should bear in mind that, although commendable, the provision of advice alone does not ensure that patients most in need of intervention actually receive any. Moreover, due to physical and psychological challenges, people with mental health illnesses may require both a tailored exercise prescription and ongoing clinical monitoring (see Chapter 9) for interventions to reduce weight.

Another common side effect of psychotropic medication is haematological and hepatic-related side effects, which we will turn to next.

Haematological and hepatic effects

A variety of blood disorders (dyscrasias) are present in people with mental health disorders and these include abnormal reduction in white blood cells (leukopenia), decrease in the number of neutrophils (neutropenia), marked reduction in leukocytes (agranulocytosis) and decrease in the number of blood platelets. These blood disorders are mainly due to the effects of psychotropic medications like antipsychotics. Other psychotropic medicines that cause blood disorders, including neutropenia and agranulocytosis, are barbiturates, benzodiazepines and antidepressants. Most blood adverse effects of medication usually disappear after the offending medicine has been stopped, although drug-induced aplastic anaemia may not resolve on drug withdrawal. Neutropenia and agranulocytosis are the most clinically important and common medicine-related blood disorders.

The mechanism by which neutropenia arises varies between medicines. Some medicines cause bone marrow suppression and others cause an increase in the peripheral destruction of white blood cells. Neutropenia due to psychotropic drug use manifests after 1–2 weeks after exposure to the offending medicine and is dependent on the duration and dosage of the medicine. Apart from antipsychotics, other known medicines that cause neutropenia include antiepileptics/ mood stabilisers, especially carbamazepine.

Agranulocytosis is life-threatening and usually appears within 3–4 weeks of initiation of the psychotropic medication. It affects people in a dose-dependent manner and affects the elderly and females more. Its mortality rate can be as high as 30%, with clozapine being the worst offending medicine, though olanzapine and phenothiazines like chlorpromazine pose a significant risk of both neutropenia and agranulocytosis. Its main clinical signs are due to secondary infection and they include fatigue, malaise, chills, weakness, cough, sore throat, fever, oral mucosal infection, pharyngitis, abscess, septicaemia and pneumonia.

If a patient who is on medication that causes blood dyscrasias develops an infection, then there is justification in suspecting that this may be due to the medication. In many instances, the patient may develop a fever which can be the only sign of an infection and therefore you should investigate all episodes of pyrexia in patients who are on these medicines. There is a need to report such occurrences promptly and as a matter of course.

It is good practice to measure the leukocyte count before treatment so that there is a baseline value in case problems occur later. The monitoring of leukocyte and neutrophil count during treatment is also important, especially in highly vulnerable groups like the elderly and females. If the leukocyte count drops significantly, then it is normal to withdraw the medicine promptly. This is because a marked drop in leukocytes may result in life-threatening infection. To counter this threat, it is normal for the patient to be administered intravenous prophylactic broad-spectrum antibacterial and antifungal therapy if the patient has low leukocyte count. As a nurse, you play a critical role in assisting in the treatment process, providing explanations to the patient and reassuring your patient where it is necessary.

Though rare, you may encounter a patient who develops neutropenia on a range of different anti-psychotics. In this case, the treatment of choice is the use of amisulpride or sulpiride, as there are no published reports of these medicines causing blood disorders. Apart from blood disorders, many psychotropic medications cause neuroleptic malignant syndrome (NMS), which we will turn to next.

Neuroleptic malignant syndrome

Case study

Greg is a 30-year-old man with a history of bipolar disorder. He was admitted to hospital in an agitated and excitable state, and as a result he was administered an intramuscular injection of haloperidol 10 mg. Six hours later, his behaviour had not improved: he was involved in a fight with another patient. He was physically restrained and administered another dose of haloperidol 10 mg and 2 mg of lorazepam. Six hours later, Greg was still restless but with a notable difference: he became increasingly confused, he showed signs of muscle rigidity, his blood pressure was 160/100 mmHg and his temperature was 39°C. The doctor was informed and he thought at the time that Greg was probably angry and frustrated because he had been physically restrained. However the doctor asked the nurses to continue to record vital signs.

The nurse called the duty doctor again when it was noticed that Greg's temperature was 40°C and his blood pressure was 90/60 mmHg. The doctor ordered a blood test. Among others, the blood tests results showed raised levels of the enzyme creatine phosphokinase (CPK): 4,731 IU/L. The rigidity, labile vital signs, confusion and raised CPK level convinced the doctor that Greg had NMS and all antipsychotics and lithium were discontinued.

NMS, like agranulocytosis, is a potentially fatal side effect of psychotropic medications and can occur any time during the course of treatment. It has a prevalence of 0.02–3% in patients taking psychotropic medications. The main symptoms of NMS are hyperthermia, muscle rigidity, mental status changes, slow movements (bradykinesia) and muscle rigidity, blood pressure instability, profuse perspiration (diaphoresis), tachycardia and altered consciousness. Greg showed most of these symptoms. There are several biochemical abnormalities that accompany NMS and these include high serum levels of the enzyme CPK, as in Greg's case. Other biochemical abnormalities include an increase in aldolase, transaminases and lactic acid dehydrogenase, reduction in serum iron concentrations, presence of metabolic acidosis and leukocytosis. Although there is ongoing debate regarding the diagnosis of NMS, there is general agreement that a patient has to show at least four of the following symptoms for the diagnosis of NMS: fever, rigidity, CPK elevation, altered consciousness and urinary incontinence. Of these, fever and rigidity must be present and Greg had both of these. Before you read further, please take part in the activity below.

Activity 8.4   *Decision making*

You notice that a patient who was previously withdrawn is unusually aggressive and restless. What action would you take and why?

Although high-potency antipsychotics like haloperidol have a strong relationship with NMS, all antipsychotics, including first- and second-generation, may precipitate the syndrome. NMS has a relationship with other medicines that block central dopamine pathways, such as metoclopramide, amoxapine, antidepressants and lithium. In rare cases, dopaminergic medicines like reserpine and tetrabenazine can provoke NMS if their cessation is abrupt.

The symptoms of NMS usually evolve over 72 hours, and if there is no treatment, they can last 10–14 days. Quite often, we miss this diagnosis during the early stages as we frequently mistake the symptoms for agitation or an increase in psychosis. NMS affects men more frequently, especially those who are agitated and had received intramuscular injection of antipsychotic medication in high and rapidly escalating doses. The concomitant use of lithium plays a part in the aetiology of NMS. It affects younger men and the mortality rate can reach 30% or higher with the use of conventional antipsychotics.

The pathophysiology of this serious condition is unknown. Multiple factors probably contribute to NMS, including dehydration, comorbid medical conditions and agitation. Other clinical, systemic and metabolic factors that have an association with NMS aetiology include agitation, poor oral intake, being physically restrained, pre-existing abnormalities of central nervous system dopamine activity or receptor function, iron deficiency, traumatic brain injury, sudden stopping of muscle relaxant (dantrolene) and psychological stress of physical disease (Al Owesie and Robert 2013).

The key to a successful intervention to prevent mortality for an individual with NMS is early detection and stopping the offending medicine. It is preferable to transfer the patient to an adult intensive care unit as soon as possible. Encouraging the patient to take fluids and electrolyte restoration is vital. Where a patient is not able to take oral fluids, you may administer fluids naso-gastrically or intravenously depending on your capability. You should encourage the patient to use a cooling fan to reduce peripheral body temperature. It is likely that the patient will be started on bromocriptine, a dopamine agonist, to improve the hypodopaminergic state which is postulated as the underlying pathophysiology of NMS. Apomorphine may have greater efficacy and faster action than bromocriptine.

Sedation

Case study

Martin is a 22-year-old university student who has a diagnosis of bipolar affective disorder. Over the past few weeks, his family and friends have noticed increasingly elated behaviour and therefore his sodium valproate and quetiapine were increased to 800 mg/day and 600 mg/day respectively. Recently he has been complaining of being unable to stay awake during the day and this is affecting his studies. His medication dose was altered to enable him to have 200 mg in the morning and 600 mg sodium valproate at night time. In respect to quetiapine, the dosage was altered so that he had 200 mg of the drug in the morning and 400 mg at night. He was encouraged to drink plenty of fluids and to exercise more.

We can define sedation as a decrease in psychomotor and cognitive performance, and it is a property of many psychotropic medicines, including antipsychotics, antidepressants, anticonvulsants, antihistamines and anxiolytics. Second-generation antipsychotics like clozapine, olanzapine and quetiapine are particularly sedative. Martin takes the second-generation antipsychotic quetiapine and a mood stabiliser. Unsurprisingly, he has experienced daytime sedation. First-generation tricyclic medicines like amitriptyline induce similar effects in patients.

Sedative medicines do not have a common pharmacology but can act on a number of inhibitory pathways in the brain, like the GABA receptor complex, histamine, adrenergic receptor and muscarinic cholinergic receptors. Quetiapine, the main medicine causing Martin's drowsiness, blocks all these receptors except GABA receptors. Sedation may be beneficial during the initial stages of treatment, particularly for patients who are highly agitated. In the long term, however, it can interfere with rehabilitation and social functioning. Sedation may have been useful during the early stages when Martin was experiencing symptoms of elation, but during the later stages it was interfering with his studies. Sedation can be difficult to distinguish from mental slowing of cognitive impairment.

The treatment of drowsiness depends on the individual's diagnosis, age, the medicine causing the drowsiness and other factors. Treatment generally involves a multifaceted plan that addresses the underlying cause and helps to minimise the abnormal drowsiness so that a person can sleep well at night, be alert during the day and lead an active, normal life. One way of achieving this is to prescribe a relatively lower dose of the medicine in the morning and a large dose at night, as in

Martin's case. A low dose in the morning is likely to minimise daytime drowsiness and a large dose at night is likely to cause drowsiness and aid sleep during the night. Other measures may include drinking extra fluids, good nutrition and short periods of sleeping, but avoiding excessive sleeping during the daytime. In some cases, the use of small amounts of caffeine can temporarily relieve drowsiness. However, ongoing or excessive use of caffeine can lead to rebound drowsiness in some people. It can also result in disturbance of sleep, causing an increase in daytime drowsiness.

Next, we turn our attention to serotonin syndrome.

Serotonin syndrome

Serotonin syndrome is a potentially life-threatening adverse reaction that may occur following therapeutic use of antidepressants or some antipsychotics. It is not an idiosyncratic medicine reaction but is predictable if there is excess serotonin in the central nervous system and this will in turn excessively stimulate the 5-HT$_2$ receptors. Numerous medicines and medicine combinations produce serotonin syndrome. Some of these medicines are most types of antidepressants, serotonin-releasing agents such as amphetamines, opioid analgesics and lithium.

Serotonin syndrome or toxicity starts within hours of ingesting the serotogenic medicines. The classic clinical features of serotonin toxicity are similar to those of NMS and include neuromuscular excitation, such as hyperreflexia, myoclonus and rigidity. Under the rubric of autonomic nervous system excitation, the patient may experience hyperthermia and tachycardia. In addition, the patient may experience an alteration in mental state such as agitation and confusion. In severe serotonin toxicity, there is a rapid rise in temperature and rigidity. Other effects can include coma, seizures and cardiac toxicity. The serotonin syndrome can easily be mistaken for other conditions such as alcohol or drug withdrawal syndrome, non-convulsive seizures and encephalitis (Buckley *et al.* 2014).

In its mild to moderate presentation, the serotonin syndrome usually resolves in 1–3 days after stopping the offending medicine. By contrast, severe serotonin toxicity is a medical emergency and the presence of severe hyperthermia and breakdown of muscle fibres (rhabdomyolysis) may complicate the condition and therefore requires intensive care support.

Supportive care mainly consists of giving a sedative to the patient if necessary and you should ensure that the patient has adequate fluid intake and monitor vital signs and urine output carefully. Preventing hyperthermia and subsequent multi-organ failure is a key goal if the patient has severe serotonin toxicity. An additional benefit of lowering temperature is that this indirectly decreases (downregulates) the activity of the 5-HT$_{2A}$ receptors in the central nervous system. You can reduce or prevent hyperthermia by using cooling fans with water sprays, ice packs or cooling blankets. Serotonin antagonists, particularly 5-HT$_{2A}$ receptor antagonists, reduce hyperthermia and other severe manifestations of serotonin toxicity. Intravenous chlorpromazine is the most commonly used serotonin antagonist, but intravenous fluid loading is essential to prevent hypotension (Isbister *et al.* 2007). From a preventive point of view, an awareness of medicines with potent serotonergic effects is the key to preventing the condition.

We now turn our attention to the serotonin discontinuation syndrome.

Serotonin discontinuation syndrome

SSRI discontinuation syndrome is a condition that can occur following the dose reduction, discontinuation or interruption of mainly SSRIs or serotonin–noradrenaline reuptake inhibitor antidepressant medications. The condition typically starts from the time of reduction in dosage or complete discontinuation, depending on the half-life of the medicine and the patient's metabolism. Currently, there is no universally acceptable definition of an SSRI syndrome. However, a discontinuation panel met in Phoenix, Arizona in 1997 and stated:

> *SSRI discontinuation symptoms . . . may emerge when an SSRI is abruptly discontinued,*
> *when doses are missed, and less frequently, during dosage reduction. In addition, the*
> *symptoms are not attributable to any other cause and can be reversed when the original agent*
> *is reinstituted, or one that is pharmacologically similar is substituted. SSRI discontinuation*
> *symptoms, in most cases, may be minimized by slowly tapering antidepressant therapy, but*
> *there have been several case reports where symptoms occurred consistently even through*
> *repeated attempts to taper therapy. Physical symptoms include problems with balance,*
> *gastrointestinal and flu-like symptoms, and sensory and sleep disturbances. Psychological*
> *symptoms include anxiety and/or agitation, crying spells, irritability and aggressiveness.*
> (Schatzberg *et al.* 1997)

Symptoms of the syndrome are many and varied, apart from the symptoms described above; these symptoms can include dizziness, electric shock-like sensations, sweating, nausea, insomnia, tremor, confusion, nightmares and vertigo. The precise mechanism of SSRI discontinuation syndrome is yet to be discovered but a putative mechanism suggests a variety of factors, including electrophysiological changes in the brain and electrophysiological changes in the body, as well as dopamine dependency, and an overexcited immune system.

SSRIs with a short half-life are more likely to cause discontinuation syndrome. Those SSRIs with a long half-life, like fluoxetine, are associated less with the syndrome. Because of its long half-life, fluoxetine has been used in the treatment of discontinuation syndrome and this can be done either by administering a single 20-mg dose of fluoxetine or by starting the patient on a low dose of fluoxetine and slowly titrating down. The discontinuation syndrome can be overcome by a gradual tapering of the medicine or prescribing a medicine with a longer half-life.

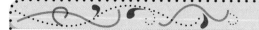

Chapter summary

The use of psychotropic medication to treat mental health disorders has revolutionised care and we now take this treatment modality for granted. In spite of its popularity, there are vexed problems. One such challenge is successful discrimination between symptoms that are intrinsic to a person's illness and potential side effects of the treatment. This may result in many side effects going unrecognised and therefore without treatment. Discussing side effects with your patient is an important part of the management process. There are many side effects of psychotropic medication but the most common tend to be extrapyramidal, metabolic, hormonal, haematological and psychic.

There are many ways of managing these side effects but basic approaches may include discontinuation of the medication and switching to a more tolerable alternative and the use of other medications to counteract the effects of the primary medicine.

Activities: brief outline answers

Activity 8.1

Age, type of medication, weight, gender, genetics and cultural values.

Activity 8.2

People going through severe dystonia also experience difficulties in swallowing (dysphagia) and therefore it is inadvisable to give oral medication.

Activity 8.3

It may be too soon to increase the dose; it is quite likely that Chris's delusions may be of a secondary nature; therefore, probe them further. Most importantly, test for prolactin levels, which may be causing him problems in terms of sexual dysfunction.

Activity 8.4

A good starting point is to speak to the patient and express your observation and take note of the patient's response. If the restlessness is due to NMS, then the patient is unlikely to give you a coherent or rational reason for the aggression and restlessness. In any event, check the medicine chart to find out what medication the patient is on and when it was last administered and route (intramuscularly or orally). Take vital signs and observe for rigidity and high temperature. If one of these is present, call the doctor straight away.

Further reading

Balon R (2007) *Practical Management of the Side Effects of Psychotropic Drugs.* New York: Marcel Dekker.

An easy-to-follow book that gives practical guidance on how to manage side effects of different psychotropic medications.

Cunnigham Owens DG (2014) *A Guide to the Extrapyramidal Side Effects of Antipsychotic Drugs.* Cambridge: Cambridge University Press.

This book discusses extrapyramidal side effects and their management in more detail.

Goldberg JF, Ernst CL (2011) *Managing Side Effects of Psychotropic Medications.* Washington, DC: American Psychiatric Publishing.

This book discusses comprehensively different types of side effects and how to manage them. Useful for prescribers and those who administer medication.

Useful websites

http://www.webmd.com/depression/managing-the-side-effects-of-antidepressants

This is a useful website that gives advice on how to manage side effects of antidepressants.

http://psychcentral.com/lib/coping-with-atypical-antipsychotic-side-effects/0002823

This website gives useful advice on how to cope with antipsychotic side effects and provides useful tips.

Chapter 9
Diet, exercise and sleep in health promotion for mental health

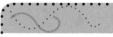

Chapter aims

By the end of the chapter, you should be able to:

*   understand and describe the importance of exercise in physical and mental health;
*   describe biological processes underpinning exercise and diet;
*   understand and describe the importance of diet in maintaining physical and mental health and well-being.

Introduction

Case study

Bill is a 46-year-old married man of African-Caribbean origin who was diagnosed with bipolar affective disorder 15 years ago. He has been taking olanzapine and lithium for the past 9 years. Although he describes his physical health as good, he is overweight (1.83 m (6 foot) tall, 93 kg (14 stone 10 lb), body mass index (BMI) 27.8 kg/m²) and on medication to control his blood pressure. There is no evidence of coronary heart disease or any family history of diabetes. However, last month his fasting glucose level was 7.1 mmol/L. Two weeks before his appointment, a random glucose test was performed and was shown to be 10.0 mmol/L. At the time of his appointment, routine laboratory results indicated slightly elevated lipids: low-density lipoprotein cholesterol 3.6 mmol/L and total cholesterol 6.2 mmol/L. Fasting glucose is 154 mg/dL. Once an avid runner, Bill has become less physically active in the past year, and his exercise consists of approximately 30 minutes of low-intensity physical activity per week.

The US Centers for Disease Control and Prevention have estimated that 80% of coronary heart disease and type 2 diabetes mellitus as well as 40% of cancers could be prevented by improving three health behaviours: eating habits, physical activity and tobacco use (US Department of Health and Human Services 2004). Physical exercise is emerging as a cost-effective way of maintaining good health and managing current physical health problems, despite drug therapy being the current gold standard for the treatment of all physical and mental health problems. This is because pharmacotherapy induces adverse side effects and has higher cost implications in comparison to physical exercise. There is growing research supporting the use of physical exercise in preventing or managing existing physical and mental health problems. Traditionally, exercise has been employed in the management of weight, but its benefits extend far beyond weight management. Current evidence shows that regular physical activity can help to reduce the risk for several physical disorders that include cardiovascular disease, diabetes, hypertension, cancer, osteoporosis, stroke and many others. Bill in the case study could benefit from physical exercise as a way of managing emerging symptoms of diabetes. Physical exercise also improves sleep, cognitive function, depression, anxiety, immune system and the fitness of both heart and lungs. Problems in these areas are common in people with mental health problems (see Chapter 1). In many respects, physical activity can be used as a distinct therapy to promote health and reduce the risk of a variety of diseases (Marcos *et al.* 2014).

This chapter starts by reviewing the importance of exercise in physical and mental disorders, and then will explore the importance of diet in maintaining good physical and mental health. Lastly, we will look at the importance of sleep in overall health and well-being.

Physical exercise and cardiovascular disease

The link between physical inactivity and cardiovascular disease is well recognised (see Chapter 4). By contrast, the benefit of exercise in the prevention and rehabilitation of those with cardiovascular problems has been well demonstrated. At least one Cochrane review has found an association between exercise and better outcome in those with cardiovascular disorders (Heran *et al.* 2011). In this systematic review of 47 studies with a total of 10,974 participants, the investigators found that exercise reduces overall cardiovascular mortality and hospital admissions. The benefits of physical exercise are mediated via several mechanisms, including the modulation of interleukin-6 (IL-6), C-reactive protein (CRP) and tumour necrosis factor-alpha (TNF-α).

IL-6 is a small protein that stimulates immune response during infection, or after tissue damage that leads to inflammation. People with cardiovascular disease or its risk factors have higher levels of these small proteins in their body, putting them at risk for developing cardiovascular disease. Another important task of IL-6 is the modulation of another inflammatory marker, CRP (see Chapter 4). Like IL-6, higher CRP levels in the body indicate the individual is at an elevated risk of developing cardiovascular disease and type 2 diabetes. Significantly, CRP concentration in the blood is the best predictor for cardiovascular disease and mortality. Physical exercise enhances immune function and exerts anti-inflammatory effects by lowering the proinflammatory cytokine IL-6 from white-fat tissues (see next section). Further, exercise lowers the levels of other proinflammatory cytokines, CRP and other chemicals whose presence is associated with cardiovascular disease. These cytokines and **biomarkers** include TNF-α (Palmefors *et al.* 2014). The TNF-α-lowering effect of physical exercise is significant, as TNF-α plays a key role in causing vascular inflammation, oxidative stress, cell death, blood vessel dysfunction and the formation of atherosclerosis. As you can see, physical exercise has a large part to play in heart health, and this is true for those with type 2 diabetes mellitus. We will go on to discuss diabetes and exercise after the first activity.

Activity 9.1 — *Critical thinking*

John is 50 years old and his BMI is 32. He had a medical check-up last week and his doctor told him that his CRP levels are higher than normal. What other factors may cause higher levels of CRP?

Type 2 diabetes and exercise

Exercise is the cornerstone of type 2 diabetes management, along with dietary and pharmacological interventions. The current recommendation is that patients with type 2 diabetes, like Bill in the case study, should perform at least 150 minutes per week of moderate-intensity aerobic exercise and should perform resistance exercise three times per week (Orozco *et al.* 2008). There are several possible ways in which exercise may improve diabetes outcome, and one mechanism involves the proinflammatory IL-6 cytokine.

Apart from its link to cardiovascular disease, IL-6 is one of several proinflammatory cytokines that play an important role in insulin resistance and type 2 diabetes. We know that people with type 2 diabetes have two or three times the normal level of circulating IL-6, but its role in glucose metabolism is currently subject to much debate (Harder-Lauridsen *et al.* 2014). However, most agree that the elevation of IL-6 plays a dual role in diabetes and this depends on where the IL-6 originates. We currently believe that, in the absence of an acute inflammation, 15–30% of circulating IL-6 levels in the body comes from white fat tissues (Bastard *et al.* 2006). Obesity enhances the production of IL-6 by the white-fat tissues. If IL-6 originates from the fat tissues, it acts as a proinflammatory cytokine which causes insulin resistance and leads to type 2 diabetes. As discussed previously, physical exercise has a lowering effect on IL-6, thus improving insulin sensitivity. Insulin sensitivity can be improved by another mechanism that involves IL-6.

Theory summary

IL-6 and exercise

During physical exercise, contracting muscle tissues produce IL-6. In contrast to IL-6 originating from the white-fat tissues, muscle-generated IL-6, called myokines, acts as anti-inflammatories or in a hormone-like manner. Myokines are small proteins that the skeletal muscles secrete during aerobic exercise and they carry out important biological functions in the muscle and other organs like the brain, heart and pancreas. Myokine biological functions include extensive anti-inflammatory action and improvement of insulin sensitivity. During muscular exercise, plasma concentration of muscle IL-6 (myokine) increases up to 100-fold and this improves insulin sensitivity, particularly in the muscles. High concentrations of muscle IL-6 may promote nutrient availability during exercise and enhance beta-cell function in the pancreas. In addition to the role of muscular IL-6 in insulin sensitivity, the production of adiponectin through exercise promotes insulin sensitivity.

The role of adiponectin in exercise

White-fat tissues secrete the protein hormone adiponectin, which regulates glucose levels as well as fatty acid breakdown. Apart from its insulin-sensitising effect, it plays a role in obesity, coronary heart disease and metabolic syndrome. High adiponectin levels also play a protective role in atherosclerosis development by suppressing inflammatory processes on the vascular endothelium. People with type 2 diabetes have low levels of adiponectin and this leads to insulin resistance. Aerobic exercise has the net effect of increasing adiponectin and therefore sensitising the person to insulin.

A systematic review of 33 randomised controlled trials on exercise showed that adiponectin increased by as much as 38% during aerobic exercise (Simpson and Singh 2008). In a separate systematic review of 47 randomised controlled trials (8,538 patients) that examined the effects of exercise on blood, the investigators found that structured exercise training that consists of aerobic exercise, resistance training, or both, has an association with glycated haemoglobin reduction in patients with type 2 diabetes. Further, structured exercise training of more than 150 minutes per week has a link with greater HbA1c reduction than that of 150 minutes or less per week. The study also found that physical activity advice was associated with lower HbA1c, but only when combined with dietary advice (Umpierre *et al.* 2011). Therefore physical exercise significantly improves symptoms in people with type 2 diabetes and there is now a recognition that it is a cornerstone for type 2 diabetes prevention and treatment. It can regulate blood sugar levels, with minimal undesirable side effects. It has benefits that extend beyond merely controlling blood glucose levels. Such benefits include improving aerobic capacity, muscular strength, body composition and endothelial function.

The use of exercise is also indicated in the treatment and management of cancer, which we will turn to next.

Cancer

Case study

Sangeeta is a 57-year-old female who suffers from schizophrenia and was diagnosed with stage 1 breast cancer 3 years ago. She had the tumour removed and completed a course of chemotherapy (cyclophos-phamide, methotrexate, 5-fluorouracil) and radiotherapy. After treatment ended, she was encouraged to take up aerobic exercise. She kept a daily log of exercise, and her Vo_{2max} increased from pretreatment. Three years after her diagnosis of breast cancer, Sangeeta reports she feels better than before.

Cancer incidence increases with advancing age and over 60% of new cancers occur in those aged 65 years or older. One factor that may contribute to this is the decline in normal function of the immune system as people get older. At Sangeeta's age, it is reasonable to assume that her immune system has declined. There are multiple age-related deficits in the immune system that may play a role in increasing incidences of cancer. These include a decrease in function of cells that detect and kill cancer (**killer cell**), impaired antigen uptake, an increase in inflammation and a decline in the number of naïve T cells responsive to evolving tumour cells (Bigley *et al.* 2013).

There is general agreement that regular physical exercise can offer protection against certain types of cancer and, in doing so, may enhance cancer prevention and treatment, particularly in the elderly, by improving adaptive immunity. In particular, aerobic fitness has a direct link with increased proportions of naïve cancer-killing T lymphocytes that can respond to ever-evolving tumours and maintain equilibrium. Sangeeta engages in aerobic exercise and this may explain why she feels healthier 3 years after treatment for cancer.

Exercise-training interventions in previously sedentary elderly people can increase T cells in the body. It may exert this protective function through prevention of visceral fat accumulation that causes inflammation. In turn, the association between chronic inflammation confirmed through elevated proinflammatory markers and cancers is well established. Therefore, the anti-inflammatory effect of exercise may also help reduce cancer risk, particularly in the elderly.

In comparison to women from the general population, the incidence of breast cancer is higher in females with schizophrenia, like Sangeeta (Bushe *et al.* 2009). Moreover, the incidence of depression and anxiety in women with breast cancer is relatively high (Lueboonthavatchai 2007). Exercise is beneficial in reducing the risk for developing breast cancer and the relative risk reduction of breast cancer for women who engage in moderate to vigorous physical activity 3–5 times per week can be up to 40% (Volaklis *et al.* 2013). In respect of breast cancer survivors, exercise training appears to be safe and improves physiological and psychological functioning. Therefore, you should encourage breast cancer survivors such as Sangeeta to participate in rehabilitation programmes which bring many physiological and psychological benefits. These include reduction in fatigue and improvements in immune function, physical body functioning, body fat composition and quality of life (Battaglini *et al.* 2014). Based on recent scientific evidence, a complete rehabilitation programme for patients with breast cancer should combine both strength and aerobic exercise in order to maximise the expected benefits.

In addition to breast cancer, multiple studies have found a correlation between frequent bouts of aerobic exercise with a reduced risk of other forms of cancer, including colorectal and prostate cancer (Lee 2003). One meta-analysis reported that high levels of physical activity may be able to reduce all-cause cancer rates by 46% (Shephard and Futcher 1997). Further, a Cochrane systematic review of 40 trials with 3,694 participants found that exercise had beneficial effects on some health-related quality-of-life markers, including cancer-specific concerns, body image/ self-esteem, emotional well-being, sexuality, sleep disturbance, social functioning, anxiety, fatigue and pain (Mishra *et al.* 2012). Overall, evidence suggests that physical exercise proffers advantages for people with cancer and this is also true for those suffering from mental health problems.

Exercise and mental health disorders

As in physical health, there is growing literature suggesting that exercise or physical activity interventions have beneficial effects across several mental health outcomes. Generally, engaging in regular physical activity has desirable health outcomes across a variety of mental health conditions, including better general health and health-related quality of life and better functional capacity in various mental health conditions that include schizophrenia, depression and anxiety (Tordeurs *et al.* 2011). We will look at depression first but, before that, let's look at the activity below.

Activity 9.2 *Evidence-based practice and research*

Alone or in a group, find out about the psychological complications of cancer treatment.

Depression and exercise

Depression is a significant public health issue and is prevalent in 10% of the population (Cassano and Fava 2002). Furthermore, depression is one-and-a-half times higher in women of childbearing age than in men and it has many consequences. Several effective treatments for depression are available but many of these have substantial pitfalls. Antidepressants are the most common form of treatment for depression; they are relatively cheap and effective but induce uncomfortable side effects, some of which can be life-threatening. These side effects include cardiotoxicity, weight gain, the serotonin syndrome, sexual dysfunction, dry mouth and urinary retention

(Mutsatsa 2011). Electroconvulsive therapy has been used in the treatment of depression since the late 1930s and is effective particularly in severe depression. It is quick-acting but its use evokes moral and ethical debates. Psychological therapies have been used since the ninth century AD and are effective and have few side effects, but they are relatively expensive and there is a long waiting list in the NHS for these therapies. Emerging evidence suggests a place for the use of exercise to improve depressive symptoms. Physical activity has consistently been shown to improve physical health, life satisfaction, cognitive functioning and psychological well-being. It compares favourably to antidepressant medications as a first-line treatment for mild to moderate depression and can improve depressive symptoms when used as an adjunct to medications (Carek *et al.* 2011). In order to understand how exercise is effective in the treatment and management of depression, we need to look at biological mechanisms that may explain depression.

Theory summary

The kynurenine pathway

Raised proinflammatory cytokines that cause neuroinflammation are well known to be involved in the development of depression or depression-like behaviours. The neuroinflammatory response causes an imbalance in tryptophan in the kynurenine pathway. The kynurenine pathway is responsible for the degradation of tryptophan, an amino acid that plays an important role in the production of serotonin. When the body comes under an immune challenge, typically from invading pathogens, it responds by increasing the amount of proinflammatory cytokines. These proinflammatory cytokines, like interferon-γ, speed up the degradation of tryptophan, a precursor to serotonin. The degradation of tryptophan to a chemical called kynurenine results in insufficient brain serotonin, a neurotransmitter that is deficient in people with depression. In addition to the role of tryptophan in depression, proinflammatory cytokines such as interferon-γ and interferon-α can directly increase serotonin reuptake from the synapse back into presynaptic neuron. This causes synaptic serotonin deficiency, leading to depression.

Exercise, and aerobic exercise in particular, reduces the level of interferon-γ and other cytokines. The reduction of interferon-γ increases tryptophan levels and this leads to increased serotonin levels in the brain. In addition to the role of the immune system in explaining depression, abnormalities in the hypothalamic–pituitary–adrenal axis play an important role in depression (Katon 2011; Muller 2014). People with major depression have elevated levels of cortisol and corticotrophic-releasing hormone and these hormones tend to revert to normal levels when a person recovers from depression.

How can physical exercise be beneficial to people with depression? Exercise reduces levels of the body's stress hormones, such as cortisol and corticotrophic-releasing hormone. Moreover, increased physical activity has a consistent association with improvement in physical health, life satisfaction, cognitive functioning and psychological well-being (Carek *et al.* 2011). This is because physical exercise promotes changes in the human brain due to increases in metabolism, oxygenation and blood flow. Exercise also controls major brain neurotransmitters that have a link to depression, such as noradrenaline, dopamine and serotonin. Other neurochemical factors released by the body during physical activities include **trophic factors**, opioids and endocannabinoids, which promote a sense of euphoria, well-being, anxiolytic effects, sedation and decreased sensitivity to pain (Dietrich and McDaniel 2004). Similar beneficial effects of exercise can be seen in schizophrenia.

Exercise and schizophrenia

Case study

Richie is a 33-year-old male who was diagnosed with schizophrenia 6 years ago. Since diagnosis, he has been admitted to hospital several times following a relapse in mental state. In the past he has said he does not like taking medication as he sees little benefit in it. He has been on several antipsychotics but his recovery has always been partial. In particular, he experiences periods of low mood, lack of motivation and poor attention and concentration. Before becoming ill, Richie used to enjoy sport but now spends most of his time asleep or indoors watching TV. As a result he has gained 8 kg (18 lb) in weight. Three months ago his older brother persuaded him to go swimming with him. Richie enjoyed swimming so much that he has been swimming regularly.

In people with schizophrenia, the beneficial effects of exercise may be greatly underappreciated. The positive effects of exercise include improved metabolic responses, as well as neuroprotection, improved quality of life, and reduction in severity of psychopathological symptoms, as in the case of Richie. With respect to the adverse metabolic effects of antipsychotic treatment, physical exercise can prevent or lessen cardiovascular disease risk factors, including elevated blood pressure, insulin resistance, glucose intolerance, elevated blood triglycerides, low high-density lipoprotein cholesterol levels and obesity, all of which are highly prevalent in patients with psychosis. Because of his sedentary lifestyle and weight gain, Richie is at risk of developing these metabolic-related side effects and therefore, physical exercise proffers advantages.

Exercise may provide direct benefit for symptoms of psychosis as well. A systematic review of 19 studies that examined the effect of exercise on symptoms of schizophrenia underlined the importance of aerobic exercise in ameliorating both positive and negative symptoms of schizophrenia. This improvement may be due to the positive effect of exercise on neurogenesis in the hippocampus region of the brain (Bernard and Ninot 2012). Exercise has beneficial effects on people suffering from dementia or having cognitive difficulties.

Exercise and dementia

As we get older, we accumulate molecular and cellular damage, which leads to a wide range of age-related pathological conditions, such as loss of protein, loss of bone mass and a concomitant increase in fat mass. This results in a growing incidence of disorders that include cognitive decline and dementia. In addition, factors like dyslipidaemia that increase as we age can lead to neurodegenerative diseases. Ageing also reduces the ability of the hypothalamus to regulate hormone secretion and this causes a reduction in the sensitivity to hormone action at the cellular level.

To compound matters further, physical inactivity at any age has a strong link with decline in some cognitive domains and cerebrovascular function, as well as an elevated risk of cerebrovascular disease and other morbidities. By contrast, physical exercise has a beneficial role on health.

Research summary

The beneficial effect of aerobic exercise on human cognitive functioning and mental well-being has been well documented (Larson et al. 2006). As early as 2003, Kramer et al. suggested that exercise could improve cognition in older adults. In particular, aerobic exercise could improve **executive function**. A systematic review of 22 studies with a total of 1,699 participants found that exercise improves or delays the onset of dementia in older adults with mild cognitive impairment. Participants showed improvement in executive function performance, attention, memory and communication after taking part in exercises. The exercise included walking, tai chi and ergonomic cycling (Ohman et al. 2014).

Exercise promotes blood flow, neurogenesis and cell proliferation in the dentate gyrus part of the hippocampus. Neurogenesis in this part of the brain has an association with improvement in cognitive function; conversely, cell loss or atrophy of the dentate gyrus of the hippocampus has an association with cognitive impairment. Furthermore, for brain cells to function appropriately, they need neurotrophic factors like **brain-derived neurotrophic factor (BDNF)**, **insulin-like growth factor** 1 and **vascular endothelial growth factor**. Exercise increases the levels of these growth factors. Several forms of exercise may be beneficial to people with mental health problems. This is particularly relevant for nurses working with older adults who may be showing signs of cognitive decline. We will now turn to different aspects of exercise but, before that, please take part in the activity below.

Activity 9.3   *Critical thinking*

Marjorie is a 76-year-old woman who is in the early stages of Alzheimer's disease. Before she was diagnosed with Alzheimer's, she led an active life and used to work for voluntary organisations when she retired. Recently her daughter has found that Marjorie gets very restless and her sleep is poor and she is reluctant to take her medication. What advice might you offer her daughter and why?

Types of exercise

At the most basic level of exercise, you could encourage your patient to take part in leisure activities that include going out to places of interest or to parks. There is evidence to suggest that exercising in natural environments offers greater benefits than exercising indoors (Pretty *et al.* 2005; Thompson *et al.* 2011), and this finding has brought about the notion of Green Exercise or Eco-therapy (Pretty *et al.* 2005). Eco-therapy is the implementation of interventions such as walking, relaxation and creative activity, aimed at improving physical, psychological and social functioning using green spaces. A systematic review of nine studies found that, compared to exercising indoors, exercising in natural environments such as parks or taking country walks is associated with greater feelings of revitalisation and positive engagement and a decrease in tension, confusion, anger, depression, as well as increased energy. The review further reported that those who participated in outdoor activities reported greater enjoyment and satisfaction and declared a greater intent to repeat the activity later. Those who participated in indoor exercise did not report the same level of satisfaction (Thompson *et al.* 2011). Exercising in green spaces may be ideal for beginners or for older persons who may be physically frail.

In formulating exercise for patients, you should take into consideration whether the patient understands the types of exercise available, the importance of exercise, and, most importantly, you need to establish the individual's fitness level to be able to tailor activities. You should provide information to patients about the benefits of exercise, and then help them decide whether they want to carry out exercise as part of a group or on their own.

Individual activities or exercises for consideration may include walking in open spaces, gardening, 1.6 km (1-mile) brisk walk, 0.8 km (0.5-mile) run, bike ride and low-impact aerobic video. Enjoyable group activities or exercises include rounders, baseball, tag, badminton, volleyball, basketball or going group bike riding.

Exercise should raise the heart rate and make you breathless. The Department of Health recommends that people should exercise for at least half an hour, five times a week. This does not have to be done all at once, as short bursts of exercise are just as beneficial. For example, instead of exercising continuously for 30 minutes you can split it into three 10-minute sessions of high-intensity exercise. Evidence suggests that very brief high-impact exercise makes the heart and lungs stronger. It burns more energy and improves insulin sensitivity (Adams 2013).

In addition to exercise, an important role in maintaining adequate physical and mental health is played by our diet.

Diet and health

Nutrition is emerging as a factor that plays a unique role in both mental and physical health. In particular the relationship between diet, brain function and the risk of mental disorders has been the subject of intense research in recent years. Restriction of calorie intake is among the most robust interventions for extending lifespan (Masoro 2005). There is sufficient evidence to support that dietary interventions such as calorie restriction have the potential to extend human lifespan significantly. In this vein, is there an ideal dietary pattern for healthy ageing, as most of the physical ailments we face are due to how our body ages? In a discouraging trend, modern societies seem to be converging on a common dietary pattern – one that is not ideal for healthy ageing. The key characteristics of this diet consist of high calorie intake, high saturated fat, sugar, and refined carbohydrates, a high intake of meat (especially red and processed meats) and a low intake of fruit, vegetables, fibre and **phytonutrients**. We often call this the 'western diet' and it is common in the UK. However, it is also a dietary pattern that, as previously mentioned, modernising societies are adopting (Willcox *et al.* 2014). This kind of dietary pattern not only leads to nutritional deficiencies but also promotes a cluster of metabolic problems, including obesity, reduced insulin sensitivity, glucose intolerance and dyslipidaemia, as well as systematic inflammation. These are all risk factors for the most common age-related diseases that include cardiovascular diseases, some cancers and type 2 diabetes. In addition, there is accumulating evidence supporting a link between diet and mental health.

Diet and mental health

There seems little doubt that dietary patterns and mental health have an intimate link with socio-economic circumstances. Moreover, the physiological responses to the consumption of energy-dense 'comfort foods' are likely to be behaviourally reinforced in people with mental health disorders. If we consider economics and convenience in people with mental health problems, the likelihood of these high-calorie foods being preferred by this population increases. Not only are fast-food outlets and convenience stores commonplace in disadvantaged areas, but outdoor advertising of high-energy, low-nutrient foods and beverages is more prevalent in such environments. How might nutrition relate to mental health?

The brain operates at a very high metabolic rate, utilising a substantial proportion of the body's energy and nutrient intake. Cellular communication in the brain (both within and between cells) is dependent upon amino acids, fats, vitamins and minerals and trace elements. The **antioxidant** defence system operates with the support of nutrient co-factors and phytochemicals are of particular relevance to mental health. A co-factor is a non-protein part of an enzyme (usually vitamin-derived) that is necessary for the enzyme to function properly. We sometimes call co-factors 'helper molecules'. Similarly, the functioning of the immune system is of substantial importance to mental health disorders and is profoundly influenced by diet and other lifestyle factors.

Neural development and repair mechanisms throughout life are also highly dependent on nutritional factors. However, the importance of nutrition as the foundation of physiological processes and a factor in promoting positive mental health has traditionally suffered from scientific neglect until recently.

A variety of epidemiological studies, including high-quality prospective studies, have linked adherence to healthy dietary patterns with lowered risk of anxiety and/or depression. The results of these studies indicate that nutrition may provide a very meaningful layer of resilience.

As a starting point, high consumption of foods that cause obesity (obesogenic foods) during the pre- and perinatal period have an association with long-term changes in neurotransmission, brain plasticity and behaviour in offspring. Further, clinical and experimental evidence indicates that an appropriate diet can reduce symptoms of depression. The neurotransmitter serotonin (5-HT), that the brain synthesises via its precursor tryptophan, plays an important role in mood alleviation, satiety and sleep regulation. As tryptophan is not naturally abundant, diets poor in this amino acid may induce depression in those who are vulnerable. A tryptophan-rich diet is important in susceptible patients, such as some females during the pre- and postmenstrual phase, in posttraumatic stress disorder, chronic pain, cancer and epilepsy (Shabbir *et al.* 2013). Foods rich in tryptophan include poultry, meat, cheese, yogurt, fish, legumes, eggs, nuts and seeds.

Further, healthy dietary patterns characterised by a high intake of vegetables, fruits, potatoes, soy products, mushrooms, seaweed and fish have recently been associated with a decreased risk of suicide (Nanri *et al.* 2013). Other specific elements that have a link with decreased risk of depressive symptoms are the consumption of green tea and coffee (Pham *et al.* 2014).

As mentioned previously, there is convincing evidence to link early nutrition to later mental health outcomes (Jacka *et al.* 2013). At the other end of the lifespan, adherence to a Mediterranean diet results in better cognitive outcomes and a reduction in the risk for dementia (Solfrizzi and Panza 2014). Results of a variety of clinical studies suggest a role for omega-3 essential fatty acids in disorders such as bipolar depression (Almeida *et al.* 2014), posttraumatic stress disorder (Matsuoka *et al.* 2010), major depression and a potential for the prevention of psychosis (Amminger *et al.* 2010).

Omega-3 essential fatty acids are responsible for maintaining cell membrane stability. They also have anti-inflammatory properties, lowering the concentration of proinflammatory cytokines, which may provoke neural damage and death. Omega fatty acids are also necessary for the synthesis of BDNF that plays a role in neurogenesis and synaptic plasticity. If the brain is lacking these components, the neurological pathways may malfunction and this may contribute to the start of certain mental health disorders. In addition to these key nutrients, our bodies need several nutrients which are essential for proper functioning, and they are summarised in Table 9.1.

Mineral	Function
Vitamin B group	Many important enzymes for the synthesis of neurotransmitters, such as serotonin and noradrenaline, depend on vitamin B_6. Vitamin B_{12} and folic acid (vitamin B_9) are a requirement in the synthesis of Sadenosylmethionine, which is essential for the metabolism of several neurotransmitters. Low levels of folic acid and B_{12} are associated with depression (Sanchez-Villegas *et al.* 2009). Deficiency in vitamin B_{12} is also associated with cardiovascular disorders but folic acid supplementation increases levels of serotonin in the brain and this is likely to alleviate depressive symptoms. Foods rich in vitamin B are pork, poultry, fish, bread, whole cereals, such as oatmeal, wheat germ and rice, eggs, vegetables and soya bean
Vitamin D	Low vitamin D levels are associated with depression and vitamin D has a neuroprotective effect against the effects of dopamine toxins such as methamphetamine. Those with low vitamin D blood serum levels are nearly twice as likely to develop depression as those who have higher levels (Jorde *et al.* 2008). Further, vitamin D is involved in neurodevelopment and modulates nerve growth factors essential for the growth and survival of many neurons in the brain. It affects the key biological functions of over 2,000 genes in the body responsible for hormone balance, cell growth and immune function. Therefore, deficiency of vitamin D can lead to a vast array of neurodevelopmental disorders like schizophrenia. Foods rich in this vitamin are fish and mushrooms, but the main source of vitamin D is exposure of the skin to sunlight

(Continued)

(Continued)

Mineral	Function
Vitamin E	Levels of vitamin E are lower in people with major depression. Vitamin E is a major fat-soluble antioxidant that plays an important part in the defence against membrane damage from reactive radicals. Foods rich in vitamin E are almonds, raw seeds, spinach, turnip greens, kale, plant oils and hazelnuts
Carnitine	Carnitine is a substance that helps the body turn fat into energy. It is made in the liver and stored in the kidneys, skeletal muscles, heart, brain and sperm. It is a powerful antioxidant that treats many conditions, including cardiovascular disorders, erectile dysfunction, kidney disease and hyperthyroidism, Alzheimer's disease and memory impairment. Foods rich in carnitine are red meat (particularly lamb), dairy products, fish, poultry, tempeh, wheat, asparagus, avocados and peanut butter
Inositol	Inositol, or vitamin B_8, is not a true vitamin because the human body has the ability to manufacture small amounts of this compound on its own. Inositol plays an important role in diverse cellular functions, such as cell growth, apoptosis, cell migration, endocytosis and cell differentiation. Several brain neurotransmitters, including serotonin and acetylcholine, require inositol for proper function. At least one meta-analytic review has confirmed the antidepressant effects of inositol (Mukai *et al.* 2014). The body produces its own inositol (small amounts) but the best sources of inositol can be found in lecithin granules, beef heart, desiccated liver, wheat germ, lecithin oil, liver, brown rice, cereals, citrus fruits, nuts, molasses, green leafy vegetables, whole-grain bread and soy flour
Selenium	Selenium is a trace element that is naturally present in many foods, and available as a dietary supplement. It is a constituent of more than two dozen selenoproteins that play critical roles in reproduction, thyroid hormone metabolism, DNA synthesis and protection from oxidative damage and infection. Skeletal muscle is the major site of selenium storage, accounting for approximately 28–46% of the total selenium pool. Considerable evidence suggests that selenium deficiency leads to depressed mood (Pasco *et al.* 2012). Seafoods and organ meats are the richest food sources of selenium. Other sources include muscle meats, cereals and other grains, and dairy products

Table 9.1: Key nutrients and their sources

Magnesium

Magnesium is the fourth most abundant mineral on earth and it is a co-factor for more than 300 metabolic reactions in the body. These reactions include protein synthesis, cellular energy production and storage, reproduction, DNA and RNA synthesis, and stabilising mitochondrial membranes. Magnesium also plays a critical role in nerve transmission, cardiac excitability, neuromuscular conduction, muscular contraction, vasomotor tone, normal blood pressure, and bone integrity, glucose and insulin metabolism. Magnesium deficiency has been associated with a number of chronic diseases, including migraine headaches, Alzheimer's disease, cerebrovascular accident, hypertension, cardiovascular disease and type 2 diabetes mellitus. Low magnesium status has an association with chronic inflammatory stress conditions.

This inflammatory response could play a role in obesity in humans because obesity has an association with chronic low-grade inflammation and low magnesium. This low-magnesium status may be due to dietary deficiencies or to drugs such as thiazide diuretics which can further worsen magnesium loss, typically through the urine. The foods highest in magnesium include unrefined grains (Solfrizzi and Panza 2014), spinach, nuts, legumes, potatoes, cereals and peanut butter.

Zinc and health

> ### Case study
>
> *Jean is a 54-year-old woman who has been suffering from depression for the past 5 years. She has taken various antidepressant medications – fluoxetine, mirtazapine and citalopram – but only experienced mild relief. She has described her appetite as 'too good'. She also had a long history of poor sleep. SpectraCell micronutrient testing revealed functional deficiencies of folic acid and zinc. She was placed on zinc supplement and encouraged to consume food rich in zinc. Follow-up SpectraCell micronutrient testing was performed 6 months later. All deficiencies were resolved and her mood had improved significantly. Her sleep pattern had improved significantly and she was waking up feeling more refreshed.*

The importance of zinc in human health was discovered in 1963. During the past 50 years, tremendous advances in zinc metabolism in humans have been observed. It is estimated that nearly a billion people worldwide are deficient in zinc. It is a trace element essential for the optimal function of the human body, especially the brain. Nearly 90% of zinc is found in the muscle and bone but very high concentrations of zinc in the brain are found in the hippocampus and amygdalar regions. Zinc is an important co-factor in more than 300 cellular enzymes, influencing various organ functions, including cell growth, apoptosis, metabolism, endocrine and immune regulation. A meta-analysis of 17 studies, with a total of 1,643 participants, found zinc concentration to be very low in depressed patients, such as in the case of Jean above. Zinc deficiency also has a link with abnormalities in antidepressant medication response (Mlyniec *et al.* 2013). This may explain why Jean was not responding to antidepressant treatment.

Zinc deficiency has been implicated in the neural function of several mental health disorders, including dementia and attention-deficit hyperactivity disorder. In physical disorders, a lack of zinc can lead to immune insufficiency, infection, diarrhoea, skin eruptions, dermatitis and poor wound healing. There are a number of studies that indicate that zinc supplementation may be helpful for people with major depression (Solati *et al.* 2014) and that it decreases the incidence of infection (Prasad 2014). Foods rich in zinc are seafood (oysters), red meat, wheat germ, spinach, cashew nuts, mushrooms and beans. Therefore it is important for patients to eat a correct diet that is nutritionally rich, such as the Mediterranean diet. But before we discuss this, please take part in the activity below.

Activity 9.4   *Evidence-based practice and research*

Jean in the case study had SpectraCell micronutrient testing. Undertake some research into this test.

The Mediterranean diet

So far, it has been clear that diet has an effect on human health and this has been confirmed by many epidemiological, population-based and randomised clinical trials. There is good evidence that a dietary pattern rich in some beneficial food groups, such as fruit, vegetables, whole grains and fish, can reduce the incidence of many physical and mental health disorders. The vast majority of studies assess single nutrients or food groups in relation to the occurrence of a particular disorder. This approach has several limitations, because food components of diet present synergistic and antagonist interactions, and in practice people consume a complex of nutrients. Therefore, over the past few years, researchers have shifted their attention from the evaluation of single nutrients to the analysis of dietary patterns as a whole. In this respect, the Mediterranean and Japanese diets are both officially on a UNESCO list of intangible cultural heritage in need of urgent safeguarding and register of best safeguarding practices.

The Mediterranean diet is a modern nutritional recommendation, originally inspired by the traditional dietary patterns of Greece, southern Italy and Spain. The principal aspects of this diet include the consumption of proportionately high olive oil, legumes, unrefined cereals, fruit and vegetables. Another aspect of the diet involves the consumption of moderate to high amounts of fish, moderate consumption of dairy products, especially cheese and yogurt, moderate wine consumption and low consumption of red meat and meat products. A meta-analysis with 4,172,412 subjects found the Mediterranean diet to be a healthy dietary pattern in terms of morbidity and mortality (Sofi *et al.* 2013). In particular, a greater adherence to the Mediterranean diet has a link to a reduction in risk of overall mortality, cardiovascular mortality, cancer incidence and mortality. Further, it has an association with reduced incidence of Parkinson's disease and Alzheimer's disease. Adherence to the Mediterranean diet was associated with perceived improvement in physical and mental health (Munoz *et al.* 2009).

Similarly, the Japanese diet proffers advantages for physical and mental health.

The Okinawa diet (Japanese)

Residents of Okinawa, the southernmost part of Japan, are known for their long average life expectancy, high numbers of people who live over the age of 100 years and a low risk of age-related diseases. Much of the longevity advantage has been attributed to a healthy lifestyle. In particular, the traditional diet, which is low in calories yet nutritionally rich with phytonutrients, antioxidants and **flavonoids**, has been particularly credited with this advantage.

If we compare diets that have an association with a reduced risk of chronic diseases, they are similar to the traditional Okinawan diet. The Okinawan diet is rich in vegetables and fruit (therefore phytonutrient- and antioxidant-rich) but low in meat, refined grains, saturated fat, sugar, salt and full-fat dairy products. Many of the characteristics of the Okinawan diet are similar to other healthy dietary patterns, such as the traditional Mediterranean diet or the modern Dietary Approaches to Stop Hypertension (DASH) diet (Shirani *et al.* 2013). Features such as the low levels of saturated fat, high antioxidant intake and low glycaemic load in these diets are likely contributory factors to a reduction in risk for cardiovascular disease, cancer and other chronic diseases. This reduction in risk is through multiple mechanisms, including a reduction in oxidative stress. A comparison of the nutrient profiles of the three dietary patterns shows that the traditional Okinawan diet is the lowest in fat intake, particularly in terms of saturated fat, and highest in carbohydrate intake. The diet consists mainly of antioxidant-rich yet calorie-poor orange-yellow root vegetables, such as sweet potatoes, and green leafy vegetables, soy products, fish and sea vegetables. Many of the components of the Okinawan diet that are consumed on a regular diet are 'functional foods' that are currently being explored for their potential health-enhancing properties (Willcox *et al.* 2009).

Below are the ten characteristics of the traditional Okinawan diet:

1. low calorie intake;
2. high consumption of vegetables (particularly root and green-yellow vegetables);
3. high consumption of legumes (mostly soybean in origin);
4. moderate consumption of fish products (more in coastal areas);
5. low consumption of meat products (mostly lean pork);
6. low consumption of dairy products;
7. low fat intake (high ratio of mono- and polyunsaturated to saturated fat);
8. emphasis on low-glycaemic-index carbohydrates;
9. high fibre intake;
10. moderate alcohol consumption.

In addition to the Mediterranean and Okinawan diet, the DASH diet is particularly recommended for reducing metabolic-related risk factors, and we will discuss this diet next.

The DASH diet

The DASH diet is, arguably, the most common diet doctors recommend to fight high blood pressure and was, in fact, originally developed by the US National Heart, Lung, and Blood Institute to do just that. The DASH dietary pattern is rich in fruit and vegetables, whole grains, low-fat dairy products, fish, poultry, beans, nuts and seeds. It also contains less sodium, sugar, fats and red meat than the usual western diet, as described above. It was designed with cardiovascular health in mind, and it is lower in cholesterol, saturated and *trans*-fatty acids. It is rich in nutrients such as potassium, magnesium, calcium, protein and fibre that are helpful for lowering blood pressure.

Research on the DASH dietary pattern has shown that not only can it lower blood pressure but it can also improve other risk factors for cardiovascular disease, such as increasing high-density lipoprotein cholesterol levels and lowering triglycerides or blood sugar. Long-term studies of the DASH dietary pattern have been associated with lower risk for hypertension and other cardiovascular diseases, diabetes and several types of cancer, among other chronic age-associated diseases (Shirani *et al.* 2013). Apart from exercise and diet, sleep plays an equally important role in the maintenance of good physical and mental health.

Sleep and health

Chronic sleep problems affect up to 80% of mental health patients, in comparison to up to 18% of adults in the general population (Krystal 2006). Sleep problems are particularly common in patients with anxiety, depression, bipolar disorder and attention-deficit hyperactivity disorder.

Traditionally, clinicians treating patients with psychiatric disorders have viewed insomnia and other sleep disorders as symptoms. But studies in both adults and children suggest that sleep problems may raise the risk for, and even directly contribute to, the development of some psychiatric disorders. Therefore, sleep plays a vital role in good health and well-being throughout life. Getting enough quality sleep at the right times can help protect mental health, physical health, quality of life and safety. This is because how people feel while awake is largely dependent on whether they have had adequate sleep or not. Certain people are prone to poor sleep and this includes those who make lifestyle choices that prevent them from getting enough sleep. Some take medicine to stay awake, abuse alcohol or drugs, or fail to leave enough time for sleep.

Some people with mental health disorders, as mentioned, usually have problems with sleep. Certain physical conditions like heart failure, heart disease, obesity, diabetes, high blood pressure, stroke or transient ischaemic attack have a link with sleep disorder. During sleep, the body works to support healthy brain function and maintain good physical health. In children and teens, sleep also helps support growth and development. By contrast, lack of sleep can create problems.

The damage from sleep deficiency can be immediate and dramatic, such as being involved in an accident, or the damage can accrue over time. For example, ongoing poor sleep puts one at risk of chronic health problems and can affect how well we think, react, work, learn and generally interact with others.

Good sleep promotes good brain function and helps the brain to prepare for the following day by forming new pathways to help one learn and remember information. Evidence shows that a good night's sleep improves learning and problem-solving skills (Taras and Potts-Datema 2005; Curcio *et al.* 2006). Sleep also helps one to pay attention, make decisions and be creative. In physical health, sleep plays an important role. It is vital for healing and repair of the heart and blood vessels. Sleep helps maintain a healthy balance of the hormones that make you feel hungry (ghrelin) or full (leptin). When one does not get enough sleep, levels of ghrelin go up and those of leptin go down. This makes one feel hungrier than when at rest. Sleep also supports healthy growth and development by triggering the body to release growth-promoting hormones in children and teenagers, which boosts muscle and mass repair.

On the other hand, sleep deficiency has a link to depression, suicide and risk-taking behaviour (Anderson and Bradley 2013). Children who are sleep-deficient may have problems getting along with others. They may feel angry and impulsive, have mood swings, feel sad or depressed, or lack motivation. They also may have problems paying attention, and they may get lower grades at school and feel stressed.

Chronic sleep deficiency has an association with elevated risk for heart and kidney disease, high blood pressure, diabetes and stroke. Sleep deficiency can increase the risk of obesity, particularly in teenagers. It can affect the way the body reacts to insulin, as sleep deficiency results in a higher than normal blood sugar level, which may increase the risk of diabetes (Kent *et al.* 2014). Ongoing sleep deficiency can change the way in which the immune system responds. For example, a person who is sleep-deficient may have trouble fighting common infections. Overall, it is clear that sleep is vital for the maintenance of good physical and mental health. Please take part in the activity below before reading further.

Activity 9.5	*Critical thinking*

John suffers from schizophrenia but he is currently in remission; however he has just informed you that he has not been able to sleep for three consecutive nights. What would be your concerns about this?

Recommended sleep hours

The amount of sleep that we need changes over the course of life. Sleep needs vary from person to person, as Table 9.2 illustrates.

Where someone consistently loses sleep or chooses to sleep less than is required, the loss of sleep is cumulative and we call this sleep debt. For example, if you lose 4 hours' sleep every night, the sleep debt will amount to 28 hours after 1 week. Napping as a way of dealing with sleeplessness provides a short-term boost in alertness and performance, but does not provide all of the other benefits of nighttime sleep. In other words, it is not really possible to make up for lost sleep.

Age	Recommended amount of sleep
Newborns	16–18 hours a day
Preschool children	11–12 hours a day
School-aged children	At least 10 hours a day
Teenagers	9–10 hours a day
Adults	7–8 hours a day

Table 9.2: Normal sleep times for different age groups

Strategies for improving sleep

There are several strategies for improving sleep and they are outlined here.

First, you may advise your patients to allow enough time to sleep. With enough sleep each night, they are likely to be happier and more productive during the day. You should advise patients to go bed and wake up at the same time every day.

The patient should keep roughly the same schedule on weeknights and weekends, limiting the difference to no more than an hour. Staying up late and sleeping in late on weekends can disrupt the body clock's sleep–wake rhythm.

You should advise the patient to take at least 1 hour before bedtime as quiet time and avoid strenuous exercise and bright artificial light, such as from a TV or computer screen. This is because the light may signal to the brain that it's time to be awake.

The patient should avoid alcoholic drinks and heavy/or large meals within a couple hours of bedtime.

Avoid nicotine (e.g. cigarettes) and caffeine such as coffee, tea and chocolate. This is because nicotine and caffeine are stimulants, and both substances can interfere with sleep. The effects of caffeine can last as long as 8 hours. So, a cup of coffee in the late afternoon can make it hard for the patient to fall asleep at night.

Advise the patient to spend time outside every day when possible and be physically active.

Advise the patient to keep the bedroom quiet, cool and dark.

A hot bath or relaxation techniques before bed are useful techniques to aid sleep.

Napping during the day may provide a boost in alertness and performance. However, if this causes problems in falling asleep at night, advise the patient to limit naps or take them earlier in the afternoon. Adults should nap for no more than 20 minutes.

Chapter summary

A majority of chronic physical disorders such as coronary heart disease, diabetes and other metabolic disorders can be prevented by embarking on three lifestyle changes: exercise, good diet and good sleep. Though exercise has traditionally been used to manage weight, there is growing research supporting the use of physical exercise in preventing or managing existing physical and mental health problems. It can help to reduce the risk of cardiovascular diseases, diabetes, hypertension, cancer, osteoporosis, stroke and many others. Physical exercise also improves sleep, cognitive function, depression, anxiety, symptoms of schizophrenia, immune system and heart and lung fitness. This is because physical exercise promotes changes in the human brain due to increases in metabolism, oxygenation and blood flow in the brain. It also controls major brain neurotransmitters that have an association with depression, such as noradrenaline, dopamine and serotonin.

Nutrition is emerging as a factor that uniquely plays a role in both mental health and physical health. In particular the relationship between diet, brain function and the risk of mental disorders has been the subject of intense research. Interventions based on calorie intake restriction are gathering momentum. These interventions have the potential to extend human lifespan significantly. Finally, sleep plays a vital role in good health and well-being throughout life. Getting enough quality sleep at the right times can help protect physical and mental health in addition to mental improvement in quality of life, and safety.

Activities: Brief outline answers

Activity 9.1

Inflammation, bacterial infection, pregnancy and burns.

Activity 9.2

Some drugs that are used in cancer treatment have been shown to cause depression. For example, treatment of cancer with the interferon cluster of drugs can cause depression.

Activity 9.3

It may be beneficial to ensure that Marjorie has some activities during the day. These may include recreational activity like a walk in the park, visiting places of interest and recreational gardening. When people exercise, it increases blood flow and cell generation, which promotes cognitive function. Further, exercise produces endocannabinoids which help to calm the individual.

Activity 9.4

SpectraCell micronutrient testing is a clinically effective diagnostic tool for the prevention and management of chronic disease conditions. It is a blood test that measures specific vitamins, minerals, antioxidants and other essential micronutrients within an individual's white blood cells. SpectraCell's tests are more clinically useful than standard serum tests. Standard tests only measure static quantities of vitamins and minerals present in serum, primarily reflecting dietary intake. But, the SpectraCell test assesses long-term intracellular requirements.

Activity 9.5

It is likely that he may be having problems. As a starting point, you may want to explore why he is not able to sleep and proffer solutions. If sleep deficiency continues, he is likely to relapse.

Further reading

Crawford C, Cadogan OU (2008) *Nutrition and Mental Health: A handbook.* Brighton: Pavilion Publishing.

Lawrence D, Bolitho S (2011) *The Complete Guide to Physical Activity and Mental Health.* London: Bloomsbury Publishing.

Useful websites

http://www.nhs.uk/Livewell/fitness/Pages/Whybeactive.aspx

A good website that explains the benefits of exercise for both physical and mental health.

http://www.nhs.uk/LiveWell/Goodfood/Pages/Goodfoodhome.aspx

This is another NHS website that gives useful information on diet and healthy living.

http://www.health.harvard.edu/newsletters/Harvard_Mental_Health_Letter/2009/July/Sleep-and-mental-health

This website gives important information on sleep and mental health.

Glossary

Adenovirus medium-sized, non-enveloped viruses that cause a wide range of illnesses, from mild respiratory infections in young children to life-threatening multi-organ disease in people with a weakened immune system

Adrenal suppression or adrenal insufficiency a condition in which the adrenal glands do not produce adequate amounts of steroid hormones, primarily cortisol; may also include impaired production of aldosterone, which regulates sodium conservation, potassium secretion and water retention

Afebrile having no fever

Agonist a chemical substance capable of activating a receptor to induce a pharmacological response

Alkaloids a group of naturally occurring chemical compounds (natural products) that contain mostly basic nitrogen atoms

Ambivalence the state of having mixed feelings or contradictory ideas about something or someone

Antecubital fossa a triangular cavity of the elbow that contains a tendon of the biceps, the median nerve and the brachial artery

Antioxidant a substance found in some foods and other products; it prevents harmful chemical reactions in which oxygen is combined with other substances

Apnoea temporary cessation of breathing, especially during sleep

Atrial fibrillation individual or uncoordinated twitching of heart muscle fibres, usually associated with heart dysfunction

Auscultatory gap a period of diminished or absent Korotkoff sounds during the manual measurement of blood pressure. The improper interpretation of this gap may lead to blood pressure-monitoring errors, namely an underestimation of systolic blood pressure and/or an overestimation of diastolic blood pressure

Biomarker measurable substance in an organism whose presence is indicative of some phenomena such as disease, infection or environmental exposure

Brain-derived neurotrophic factor (BDNF) acts as a fertiliser of the brain's neurons, making them grow more quickly and develop stronger connections

Bronchoconstriction the tightening and narrowing of airway muscles resulting in airflow blockage. Along with inflammation of the airways, it leads to symptoms such as coughing, wheezing and shortness of breath

Cardiac arrhythmias abnormal heart beats, usually caused by an electrical 'short circuit' in the heart

Cardiac myopathy a weakening of or other problem with the heart muscle. It often occurs when the heart cannot pump as well as it should, or with other heart function problems. Most patients with cardiomyopathy have heart failure

Change talk the client's mention and discussion of his or her desire, ability, reason and need to change behaviour and commitment to changing. The point here is that, when people themselves talk about change, they are more likely to change than if someone else, such as a nurse or relative, talks about it

CK or CK-MB tests a cardiac marker used to assist the diagnosis of an acute myocardial infarction. It measures the blood level of the enzyme phosphocreatine kinase

Coagulability the ability to coagulate, that is, to change from liquid into a solid or semi-solid mass, as in the case of blood

Coin lesions a round, well-circumscribed nodule in a lung that is seen on X-ray as a shadow the size and shape of a coin

Coronavirus species in the genera of virus belonging to one of two subfamilies, Coronavirinae and Torovirinae. They are found in the nasal cavities, infect the upper respiratory tract and can also cause gastroenteritis

Cytokines small proteins released by cells that have a specific effect on communication between cells or on the behaviour of cells

Diagnostic overshadowing the process of over-attributing a patient's symptoms to a particular condition, resulting in key comorbid conditions being undiagnosed and untreated. For example, symptoms of physical illness may be attributed to the service user's mental illness

Diaphoresis artificially induced profuse perspiration

Diastolic blood pressure the pressure in the arteries when the heart muscle is resting between beats and refilling with blood. It is the bottom number in blood pressure measurement, and is also the lower of the two numbers

Dynamic equilibrium exists when the rate of the forward reaction is equal to the reverse reaction

Dyslipidaemia a metabolic disorder of fat-like substance (lipoprotein) that may result in overproduction or deficiency of these lipoproteins. It is typically shown by an increase in the total cholesterol, the 'bad' low-density lipoprotein (LDL) cholesterol and the triglyceride concentrations, and a decrease in the 'good' high-density lipoprotein (HDL) cholesterol concentration in the blood

Executive function a set of mental processes that help connect past experience with present action. People use executive function to perform activities such as planning, organising, strategising, paying attention to and remembering details and managing time and space

Fasciculations involuntary contractions or twitching of groups of muscle fibres. It can occur in normal individuals without an associated disease or condition, or it can occur as a result of illness, such as muscle cramps, nerve disease or metabolic imbalance

Fibrinolytic substances which prevent blood clots from growing and becoming problematic

Flavonoid organic compound or biological pigment containing no nitrogen, found in many plants

Gastro-oesophageal reflux disease a condition in which the stomach contents leak backwards from the stomach into the oesophagus. This action can irritate the oesophagus, causing heartburn and other symptoms

Genome-wide association studies an examination of the many common genetic variants in individuals to associate any variants with a trait

Glossitis an inflammation of the tongue causing swelling, change in colour and a smooth appearance on the surface

Glucokinase an enzyme that facilitates phosphorylation of glucose to glucose-6-phosphate. It occurs in cells in the liver, pancreas, gut and brain of humans and most other vertebrates. In each of these organs it plays an important role in the regulation of carbohydrate metabolism by acting as a glucose sensor, triggering shifts in metabolism or cell function in response to rising or falling levels of glucose, such as occur after a meal or when fasting

Hyperglycaemia excess glucose in the blood stream, often associated with diabetes mellitus

Hyperinsulinaemia excess insulin circulating in the blood relative to the level of glucose

Hyperlipidaemia an abnormally elevated level of lipids (fats) in the blood plasma. It is a significant risk factor for coronary artery disease

Hyper-reflexia an exaggerated response of the deep tendon reflexes, usually resulting from injury to the central nervous system or metabolic disease

Hypertension abnormally high blood pressure

Hyperviscosity syndrome a group of symptoms triggered by increased thickening of the blood

Hypoglycaemia deficiency of glucose in the blood stream

Hypokalaemia deficiency of potassium in the blood stream

Insulin-like growth factor proteins similar to insulin that are secreted either during fetal development or during childhood and that mediate growth hormone activity

Ischaemic heart disease a disease of the blood vessels supplying the heart muscles with oxygen that causes temporary strain on the heart or even permanent damage to the muscle

Killer cell (T cell, natural killer cell) a white blood cell (lymphocyte) with cytotoxic activity

Korotkoff sound the sounds we listen for when we take blood pressure using a non-invasive procedure. They are named after Nikolai Korotkoff, a Russian doctor who discovered them in 1905

Lactated Ringer's solution a sterile, non-pyrogenic solution for fluid and electrolyte replenishment in single-dose containers for intravenous administration

Mallory–Weiss tears severe and prolonged vomiting can result in lacerations (tears) in the lining of the oesophagus. Most tears heal within a few days without treatment, but Mallory–Weiss tears can cause significant bleeding. Depending on the severity of the laceration, surgery may be required to repair the damage

Maturity-onset diabetes of the young (MODY) a rare form of diabetes which is different from both type 1 and type 2 diabetes, and runs strongly in families. MODY is caused by a mutation (or change) in a single gene. If a parent has this gene mutation, any child has a 50% chance of inheriting it from the parent

Maximal pulsation the place where the apical pulse is palpated as strongest

Metabolic acidosis an abnormally high acidity in the body during the metabolism of sugar

Metabolic syndrome cluster of biochemical and physiological abnormalities associated with the development of cardiovascular disease and type 2 diabetes

Metapneumovirus a virus family that is the second most common cause, after respiratory syncytial virus, of lower respiratory infection in young children

Monopharmacy the use of a single drug to treat a specific disorder or symptoms

Mucociliary clearance the self-clearing mechanism of the bronchi using the cilia

Oxidative stress essentially an imbalance between the production of molecules that cause damage to cells in our bodies and the ability of the body to counteract or detoxify their harmful effects through neutralisation by antioxidants

Pericellular fibrosis the formation of excess fibrous connective tissue around cells in a reparative or reactive process. This can be a reactive, benign or pathological state

Phospholipid a class of fats (lipids) that are a major component of all cell membranes as they can form lipid bilayers

Phytonutrients (phytochemicals) chemical compounds that occur naturally in plants. Some are responsible for colour and other sense-stimulating properties, such as the deep purple of blueberries and the smell of garlic. There may be as many as 4,000 different phytochemicals having the potential to affect positively recovery from diseases such as cancer, stroke or metabolic syndrome

Pneumomediastinum air in the mediastinum. The mediastinum is the space in the middle of the chest, between the lungs

Pneumothorax the presence of air or gas in the cavity between the lungs and the chest wall, causing lung collapse

Polypharmacy the simultaneous use of multiple drugs to treat a single ailment or condition

Proinflammatory markers proteins that promote inflammation

Pulmonary oedema an excess collection of watery fluid in the air sacs of the lungs, making it difficult for the individual to breathe

Pulse pressure difference between systolic and diastolic blood pressure

Regenerative nodules a form of non-neoplastic nodule that arises in a cirrhotic liver

Respiratory syncytial virus (RSV) a virus that causes infections of the lungs and respiratory tract. It is common in children and can also infect adults

Rhabdomyolysis the breakdown of muscle fibres that leads to the release of muscle fibre contents (myoglobin) into the blood stream. Myoglobin is harmful to the kidney and often causes kidney damage

Rhinovirus the most common viral infective agents in humans and the predominant cause of the common cold. They flourish in temperatures between 33 and 35°C, the temperatures found in the nose

Secondary delusions false beliefs held in spite of invalidating evidence but that are, at least in principle, understandable in the context of a person's life history, personality, mood state or presence of other psychopathology. For example, a person becomes depressed, suffers very low mood and self-esteem, and subsequently believes that s/he is responsible for some terrible crime which s/he did not commit

Serum myoglobin test blood test used to measure the levels of myoglobin in the blood stream

Socratic questioning disciplined questioning that can be used to pursue thought in many directions and for many purposes, including to explore complex ideas, to get to the truth of things, to open up issues and problems, to uncover assumptions, to analyse concepts, and to distinguish what we know from what we do not know

Stomatitis soreness or inflammation in the mouth. This can be in the cheeks, gums, inside of the lips, or on the tongue. There are two main forms of stomatitis: herpes stomatitis and aphthous stomatitis. Both forms usually occur more often in children and teens

Systolic pressure the pressure in the arteries when the heart muscle contracts. It is indicated by the top number in blood pressure measurement and is usually the higher of the two numbers

Triglyceride a naturally occurring ester consisting of glycerol and three fatty acids

Trophic factors chemicals that are essential for the growth and survival of the neuron, synapsing with it with other neurons

Troponin test measures the levels of troponin in the blood. Troponins are proteins released when the heart muscle has been damaged, such as occurs with a heart attack. The more damage there is to the heart, the greater the amount of troponin in the blood

Variance the fact or quality of being different, divergent or inconsistent

Vascular endothelial growth factor a signal protein produced by cells that stimulates the formation of new blood vessels. It is part of the system that restores the oxygen supply to tissues when blood circulation is inadequate

Ventricular fibrillation a condition in which there is uncoordinated contraction of the cardiac muscle of the ventricles in the heart, making them quiver rather than contract properly

Wernicke's encephalopathy a neurological disorder caused by thiamine deficiency, typically from chronic alcoholism or persistent vomiting, and marked by mental confusion, abnormal eye movements and unsteady gait

Wernicke–Korsakoff a brain disorder due to thiamine (vitamin B_1) deficiency

References

Adam SK, Osborne S (1997) *Critical Care Nursing*. Oxford: Oxford University Press.

Adams OP (2013) The impact of brief high-intensity exercise on blood glucose levels. *Diabetes Metab. Syndr. Obes.* **6**, 113–122.

Adsett J, Hickey A, Nagle A, Mudge A (2013) Implementing a community-based model of exercise training following cardiac, pulmonary, and heart failure rehabilitation. *J Cardiopulm. Rehabil. Prev.* **33**, 239–243.

Ajzen I (1991) The theory of planned behavior. *Organ. Behav. Hum. Decision Processes* **50**, 179–182.

Al Owesie RM, Robert AA (2013) Delirium followed by neuroleptic malignant syndrome in rehabilitation setting. Is it anger reaction before discharge? *Pan Afr. Med. J.* **15**, 26.

Almeida OP, Yeap BB, Hankey GJ, Golledge J, Flicker L (2014) HDL cholesterol and the risk of depression over 5 years. *Mol. Psychiatry* **19**, 637–638.

Amlani S, Nadarajah T, McIvor RA (2011) Montelukast for the treatment of asthma in the adult population. *Expert Opin. Pharmacother.* **12**, 2119–2128.

Amminger GP, Schafer MR, Papageorgiou K, Klier CM, Cotton SM, Harrigan SM, Mackinnon A, McGorry PD, Berger GE (2010) Long-chain omega-3 fatty acids for indicated prevention of psychotic disorders: a randomized, placebo-controlled trial. *Arch. Gen. Psychiatry* **67**, 146–154.

Anderson KN, Bradley AJ (2013) Sleep disturbance in mental health problems and neurodegenerative disease. *Nat. Sci. Sleep* **5**, 61–75.

Anderson P, Baumberg B (2006) *Alcohol in Europe: A public health perspective*. London: UK Institute of Alcohol Studies.

Arana GW (2000) An overview of side effects caused by typical antipsychotics. *J. Clin. Psychiatry* **61** (Suppl 8), 5–11.

Arking DE, Chakravarti A (2009) Understanding cardiovascular disease through the lens of genome-wide association studies. *Trends Genet.* **25**, 387–394.

Ashton CH (2001) Pharmacology and effects of cannabis: a brief review. *Br. J. Psychiatry* **178**, 101–106.

Asmal L, Flegar SJ, Wang J, Rummel-Kluge C, Komossa K, Leucht S (2013) Quetiapine versus other atypical antipsychotics for schizophrenia. *Cochrane Database Syst. Rev.* **11**, CD006625.

Baldacchino A, Balfour DJ, Passetti F, Humphris G, Matthews K (2012) Neuropsychological consequences of chronic opioid use: a quantitative review and meta-analysis. *Neurosci. Biobehav. Rev.* **36**, 2056–2068.

Bandura A (1977a) *Social Learning Theory*. Englewood Cliffs: Prentice Hall.

Bandura A (1977b) Self-efficacy: toward a unifying theory of behavioral change. *Psychol. Rev.* **84**, 191–215.

Bandura A (1991) Social cognitive theory of self-regulation. *Organiz. Behav. Hum. Decision Processes* **50**, 248–287.

Bao YP, Liu ZM, Epstein DH, Du C, Shi J, Lu L (2009) A meta-analysis of retention in methadone maintenance by dose and dosing strategy. *Am. J. Drug Alcohol Abuse* **35**, 28–33.

Barnes TR (1989) A rating scale for drug-induced akathisia. *Br. J. Psychiatry* **154**, 672–676.

Barnes TR, Braude WM (1985) Akathisia variants and tardive dyskinesia. *Arch. Gen. Psychiatry* **42**, 874–878.

Bastard JP, Maachi M, Lagathu C, Kim MJ, Caron M, Vidal H, Capeau J, Feve B (2006) Recent advances in the relationship between obesity, inflammation, and insulin resistance. *Eur. Cytokine Netw.* **17**, 4–12.

Battaglini CL, Mills RC, Phillips BL, Lee JT, Story CE, Nascimento MG, Hackney AC (2014) Twenty-five years of research on the effects of exercise training in breast cancer survivors: a systematic review of the literature. *World J. Clin. Oncol.* **5**, 177–190.

Becker MH, Drachman RH, Kirscht JP (1974) A new approach to explaining sick-role behavior in low-income populations. *Am. J. Public Health* **64**, 205–216.

Ben AM, Potvin S (2007) Cannabis and psychosis: what is the link? *J Psychoactive Drugs* **39**, 131–142.

Bennett J, Done J, Hunt B (1995) Assessing the side-effects of antipsychotic drugs: a survey of CPN practice. *J. Psychiatr. Ment. Health Nurs.* **2**, 177–182.

Benowitz NL (1988) Drug therapy. Pharmacologic aspects of cigarette smoking and nicotine addition. *N. Engl. J. Med* **319**, 1318–1330.

Benowitz NL (2009) Pharmacology of nicotine: addiction, smoking-induced disease, and therapeutics. *Annu. Rev. Pharmacol. Toxicol.* **49**, 57–71.

Bernard C, Hoff HE, Guillemin R, Guillemin L (translators) (1974) *Lectures on the Phenomena of Life Common to Animals and Plants.* Springfield, IL, USA: Charles C Thomas.

Bernard P, Ninot G (2012) Benefits of exercise for people with schizophrenia: a systematic review. *Encephale* **38**, 280–287.

Bigley AB, Spielmann G, LaVoy EC, Simpson RJ (2013) Can exercise-related improvements in immunity influence cancer prevention and prognosis in the elderly? *Maturitas* **76**, 51–56.

Blitz M, Blitz S, Hughes R, Diner B, Beasley R, Knopp J, Rowe BH (2005) Aerosolized magnesium sulfate for acute asthma: a systematic review. *Chest* **128**, 337–344.

Blows WT (2012) *The Biological Basis of Clinical Observations.* London: Routledge.

Bosch J, Gerstein HC, Dagenais GR, Diaz R, Dyal L, Jung H, Maggiono AP, Probstfield J, Ramachandran A, Riddle MC, Ryden LE, Yusuf S (2012) n-3 fatty acids and cardiovascular outcomes in patients with dysglycemia. *N. Engl. J. Med.* **367**, 309–318.

Boydell J, van OJ, Caspi A, Kennedy N, Giouroukou E, Fearon P, Farrell M, Murray RM (2006) Trends in cannabis use prior to first presentation with schizophrenia, in South-East London between 1965 and 1999. *Psychol. Med.* **36**, 1441–1446.

Braunwald E (1997) *Heart Disease: A textbook of cardiovascular medicine.* Philadelphia: Saunders.

Brimblecombe N (2006) *From Values to Action: The chief nursing officer's report on mental health nursing.* London: Department of Health.

British Thoracic Society (2009) *British Guideline on the Management of Asthma: A national clinical guideline.* Available online at: https://www.brit-thoracic.org.uk/document-library/clinical-information/asthma/btssign-asthma-guideline-2009 (accessed 15 December 2014).

Brown AD, Barton DA, Lambert GW (2009) Cardiovascular abnormalities in patients with major depressive disorder: autonomic mechanisms and implications for treatment. *CNS Drugs* **23**, 583–602.

Brown S, Birtwistle J, Roe L, Thompson C (1999) The unhealthy lifestyle of people with schizophrenia. *Psychol. Med.* **29**, 697–701.

Buckley NA, Dawson AH, Isbister GK (2014) Serotonin syndrome. *BMJ* **348**, g1626.

Buckley PF, Miller DD, Singer B, Arena J, Stirewalt EM (2005) Clinicians' recognition of the metabolic adverse effects of antipsychotic medications. *Schizophr. Res.* **79**, 281–288.

Bushe CJ, Bradley AJ, Wildgust HJ, Hodgson RE (2009) Schizophrenia and breast cancer incidence: a systematic review of clinical studies. *Schizophr. Res.* **114**, 6–16.

Butterworth RF (1995) Pathophysiology of alcoholic brain damage: synergistic effects of ethanol, thiamine deficiency and alcoholic liver disease. *Metab. Brain Dis.* **10**, 1–8.

Cahill K, Stead LF, Lancaster T (2012) Nicotine receptor partial agonists for smoking cessation. *Cochrane Database. Syst. Rev.* **4**, CD006103.

Cancer Research UK. *Smoking and Cancer: What's in a cigarette?* Available online at: http://www.cancerresearchuk.org/cancer-info/healthyliving/smoking-and-cancer/whats-in-a-cigarette/smoking-and-cancer-whats-in-a-cigarette (accessed 15 December 2014).

Carek PJ, Laibstain SE, Carek SM (2011) Exercise for the treatment of depression and anxiety. *Int. J. Psychiatry Med.* **41**, 15–28.

Casagrande SS, Anderson CA, Dalcin A, Appel LJ, Jerome GJ, Dickerson FB, Gennusa JV, Daumit GL (2011) Dietary intake of adults with serious mental illness. *Psychiatr. Rehabil. J.* **35**, 137–140.

Cassano P, Fava M (2002) Depression and public health: an overview. *J. Psychosom. Res.* **53**, 849–857.

Chang CC, Cheng AC, Chang AB (2012) Over-the-counter (OTC) medications to reduce cough as an adjunct to antibiotics for acute pneumonia in children and adults. *Cochrane Database Syst. Rev.* **2**, CD006088.

Chen JJ, Ondo WG, Dashtipour K, Swope DM (2012) Tetrabenazine for the treatment of hyperkinetic movement disorders: a review of the literature. *Clin. Ther.* **34**, 1487–1504.

Chen YH, Lee HC, Lin HC (2009) Prevalence and risk of atopic disorders among schizophrenia patients: a nationwide population based study. *Schizophr. Res.* **108**, 191–196.

Chou FH, Tsai KY, Chou YM (2013) The incidence and all-cause mortality of pneumonia in patients with schizophrenia: a nine-year follow-up study. *J. Psychiatr. Res.* **47**, 460–466.

Chwastiak LA, Rosenheck RA, McEvoy JP, Stroup TS, Swartz MS, Davis SM, Lieberman JA (2009) The impact of obesity on health care costs among persons with schizophrenia. *Gen. Hosp. Psychiatry* **31**, 1–7.

Clarke JG, Stein LA, Martin RA, Martin SA, Parker D, Lopes CE, McGovern AR, Simon R, Roberts M, Friedman P, Bock B (2013) Forced smoking abstinence: not enough for smoking cessation. *J.A.M.A. Intern. Med.* 1–6.

Collins R, Peto R, Baigent C, Sleight P (1997) Aspirin, heparin, and fibrinolytic therapy in suspected acute myocardial infarction. *N. Engl. J. Med.* **336**, 847–860.

Conner M, Norman P (2005) *Predicting Health Behaviour*. New York: McGraw-Hill International.

Connolly M, Kelly C (2005) Lifestyle and physical health in schizophrenia. *Adv. Psychiatr. Treat.* **11**, 125–132.

Copeland WE, Shanahan L, Worthman C, Angold A, Costello EJ (2012) Generalized anxiety and C-reactive protein levels: a prospective, longitudinal analysis. *Psychol. Med.* **42**, 2641–2650.

Critchley J, Capewell S (2004) Smoking cessation for the secondary prevention of coronary heart disease. 11. *Cochrane Database Syst. Rev.* CD003041.

Curcio G, Ferrara M, De GL (2006) Sleep loss, learning capacity and academic performance. *Sleep Med. Rev.* **10**, 323–337.

Daumit GL, Clark JM, Steinwachs DM, Graham CM, Lehman A, Ford DE (2003) Prevalence and correlates of obesity in a community sample of individuals with severe and persistent mental illness. *J. Nerv. Ment. Dis.* **191**, 799–805.

de Hert KL, Merchant AT, Pogue J, Anand SS (2007) Waist circumference and waist-to-hip ratio as predictors of cardiovascular events: meta-regression analysis of prospective studies. *Eur. Heart J.* **28**, 850–856.

de Hert M, van Winkel R, Van Eyck D, Hanssens L, Wampers M, Scheen A, Peuskens J (2006) Prevalence of diabetes, metabolic syndrome and metabolic abnormalities in schizophrenia over the course of the illness: a cross-sectional study. *Clin. Pract. Epidemiol. Ment. Health* **2**, 14.

de Onis M, Habicht JP (1996) Anthropometric reference data for international use: recommendations from a World Health Organization Expert Committee. *Am. J. Clin. Nutr.* **64**, 650–658.

DeFronzo RA (2010) Insulin resistance, lipotoxicity, type 2 diabetes and atherosclerosis: the missing links. The Claude Bernard Lecture 2009. *Diabetologia* **53**, 1270–1287.

Degenhardt L, Baxter AJ, Lee YY, Hall W, Sara GE, Johns N, Flaxman A, Whiteford HA, Vos T (2014a) The global epidemiology and burden of psychostimulant dependence: findings from the Global Burden of Disease Study 2010. *Drug Alcohol Depend.* **137**, 36–47.

Degenhardt L, Charlson F, Mathers B, Hall WD, Flaxman AD, Johns N, Vos T (2014b) The global epidemiology and burden of opioid dependence: results from the Global Burden of Disease 2010 study. *Addiction* **109**, 1320–1333.

Department of Health (1999a) *Effective Care Coordination in Mental Health Services: Modernising the Care Program Approach*. Available online at: http://www.rcn.org.uk/__data/assets/pdf_file/0003/522750/careprogapproachpdf.pdf (accessed 15 December 2014).

Department of Health (1999b) *Framework for Mental Health: Modern standards and service models*. London: Department of Health.

Department of Health (2007) *National Treatment Agency for Substance Misuse, Reducing Drug Related Harm: An Action Plan*. Available online at: http://www.dh.gov.uk/en/Publicationsandstatistics/Publications/ PublicationsPolicyAndGuidance/DH_074850 (accessed 15 December 2014).

Department of Health (2011) *Outcomes Strategy for Chronic Obstructive Pulmonary Disease (COPD) and Asthma in England*. London: Department of Health.

Deurenberg P, Deurenberg YM, Wang J, Lin FP, Schmidt G (1999) The impact of body build on the relationship between body mass index and percent body fat. *Int. J. Obes. Relat. Metab. Disord.* **23**, 537–542.

Di MF, Verga M, Santus P, Giovannelli F, Busatto P, Neri M, Girbino G, Bonini S, Centanni S (2010) Close correlation between anxiety, depression, and asthma control. *Respir. Med.* **104**, 22–28.

Dietrich A, McDaniel WF (2004) Endocannabinoids and exercise. *Br. J. Sports Med.* **38**, 536–541.

Dipasquale S, Pariante CM, Dazzan P, Aguglia E, McGuire P, Mondelli V (2013) The dietary pattern of patients with schizophrenia: a systematic review. *J. Psychiatr. Res.* **47**, 197–207.

Doyle TA, de GM, Harris T, Schwartz F, Strotmeyer ES, Johnson KC, Kanaya A (2013) Diabetes, depressive symptoms, and inflammation in older adults: Results from the Health, Aging, and Body Composition Study. *J. Psychosom. Res.* **75**, 419–424.

Drummond DC (2004) An alcohol strategy for England: the good, the bad and the ugly. *Alcohol Alcohol* **39**, 377–379.

Evins AE, Cather C, Deckersbach T, Freudenreich O, Culhane MA, Olm-Shipman CM, Henderson DC, Schoenfeld DA, Goff DC, Rigotti NA (2005) A double-blind placebo-controlled trial of bupropion sustained-release for smoking cessation in schizophrenia. *J. Clin. Psychopharmacol.* **25**, 218–225.

Faggiano F, Vigna-Taglianti F, Versino E, Lemma P (2003) Methadone maintenance at different dosages for opioid dependence. *Cochrane Database Syst. Rev.* CD002208.

Farrelly S, Harris MG, Henry LP, Purcell R, Prosser A, Schwartz O, Jackson H, McGorry PD (2007) Prevalence and correlates of comorbidity 8 years after a first psychotic episode. *Acta Psychiatr. Scand.* **116**, 62–70.

Fauci AS, Brauwald E, Kasper DL, Longo DL (2008) *Harrison's Principles of Internal Medicine*. London: McGraw Hill.

Forey BA, Thornton AJ, Lee PN (2011) Systematic review with meta-analysis of the epidemiological evidence relating smoking to COPD, chronic bronchitis and emphysema. *BMC Pulm. Med.* **11**, 36.

Fox BD, Kahn SR, Langleben D, Eisenberg MJ, Shimony A (2012) Efficacy and safety of novel oral anticoagulants for treatment of acute venous thromboembolism: direct and adjusted indirect meta-analysis of randomised controlled trials. *BMJ* **345**, e7498.

Frank AF, Gunderson JG (1990) The role of the therapeutic alliance in the treatment of schizophrenia. Relationship to course and outcome. *Arch. Gen. Psychiatry* **47**, 228–236.

Frank E (1997) Enhancing patient outcomes: treatment adherence. *J. Clin. Psychiatry* **58** (Suppl 1), 11–14.

French JK, Hyde TA, Patel H, Amos DJ, McLaughlin SC, Webber BJ, White HD (1999) Survival 12 years after randomization to streptokinase: the influence of thrombolysis in myocardial infarction flow at three to four weeks. *J. Am. Coll. Cardiol.* **34**, 62–69.

Freud S (1912) A dinâmica da transferência. In: *Edição Standard Brasileira das Obras Completas*, vol. 12. Rio de Janeiro: Imago (1976), pp. 131–143.

Froguel P, Guy-Grand B, Clement K (2000) Genetics of obesity: towards the understanding of a complex syndrome. *Presse Med.* **29**, 564–571.

Fu SS, McFall M, Saxon AJ, Beckham JC, Carmody TP, Baker DG, Joseph AM (2007) Post-traumatic stress disorder and smoking: a systematic review. *Nicotine Tob. Res.* **9**, 1071–1084.

Gabbard GO (2005) Does psychoanalysis have a future? Yes. *Can. J. Psychiatry* **50**, 741–742.

Gao K, Kemp DE, Ganocy SJ, Gajwani P, Xia G, Calabrese JR (2008) Antipsychotic-induced extrapyramidal side effects in bipolar disorder and schizophrenia: a systematic review. *J. Clin. Psychopharmacol.* **28**, 203–209.

Garvey JL (2006) ECG techniques and technologies. *Emerg. Med. Clin. North Am.* **24**, 209–225, viii.

George TP, Ziedonis DM, Feingold A, Pepper WT, Satterburg CA, Winkel J, Rounsaville BJ, Kosten TR (2000) Nicotine transdermal patch and atypical antipsychotic medications for smoking cessation in schizophrenia. *Am. J. Psychiatry* **157**, 1835–1842.

Goldberg JF, Ernst CL (2012) *Managing the Side Effects of Psychotropic Medications.* Arlington, VA: American Psychiatric Association.

Gossop M (1990) The development of a Short Opiate Withdrawal Scale (SOWS). *Addict. Behav.* **15**, 487–490.

Goyal S, Agrawal A (2013) Ketamine in status asthmaticus: a review. *Ind. J. Crit. Care Med.* **17**, 154–161.

Grattan A, Sullivan MD, Saunders KW, Campbell CI, Von Korff MR (2012) Depression and prescription opioid misuse among chronic opioid therapy recipients with no history of substance abuse. *Ann. Fam. Med.* **10**, 304–311.

Grech A, van OJ, Jones PB, Lewis SW, Murray RM (2005) Cannabis use and outcome of recent onset psychosis. *Eur. Psychiatry* **20**, 349–353.

Green B, Young R, Kavanagh D (2005) Cannabis use and misuse prevalence among people with psychosis. *Br. J. Psychiatry* **187**, 306–313.

Groop L (2000) Genetics of the metabolic syndrome. *Br. J. Nutr.* **83** (Suppl 1), S39–S48.

Guy W (1976) *Assessment Manual for Psychopathology*, revised edn. Washington, DC: Department of Education, Health and Welfare, pp. 534–537.

Haffner SM (2004) Dyslipidemia management in adults with diabetes. *Diabetes Care* **27** (Suppl 1), S68–S71.

Hallak JE, Dursun SM, Bosi DC, de Macedo LR, Machado-de-Sousa JP, Abrao J, Crippa JA, McGuire P, Krystal JH, Baker GB, Zuardi AW (2011) The interplay of cannabinoid and NMDA glutamate receptor systems in humans: preliminary evidence of interactive effects of cannabidiol and ketamine in healthy human subjects. *Prog. Neuropsychopharmacol. Biol. Psychiatry* **35**, 198–202.

Halstead SM, Barnes TR, Speller JC (1994) Akathisia: prevalence and associated dysphoria in an in-patient population with chronic schizophrenia. *Br. J. Psychiatry* **164**, 177–183.

Hansen TE, Casey DE, Hoffman WF (1997) Neuroleptic intolerance. *Schizophr. Bull.* **23**, 567–582.

Harder-Lauridsen NM, Krogh-Madsen R, Holst JJ, Plomgaard P, Leick L, Pedersen BK, Fischer CP (2014) Effect of IL-6 on the insulin sensitivity in patients with type 2 diabetes. *Am. J. Physiol. Endocrinol. Metab.* **306**, E769–E778.

Harrison I, Joyce EM, Mutsatsa SH, Hutton SB, Huddy V, Kapasi M, Barnes TR (2008) Naturalistic follow-up of co-morbid substance use in schizophrenia: the West London first-episode study. *Psychol. Med.* **38**, 79–88.

Hasnain M, Fredrickson SK, Vieweg WV, Pandurangi AK (2010) Metabolic syndrome associated with schizophrenia and atypical antipsychotics. *Curr. Diab. Rep.* **10**, 209–216.

Haupt DW, Newcomer JW (2002) Abnormalities in glucose regulation associated with mental illness and treatment. *J. Psychosom. Res.* **53**, 925–933.

Hazari N, Kate N, Grover S (2013) Clozapine and tardive movement disorders: a review. *Asian J. Psychiatr.* **6**, 439–451.

Heinrich J (2011) Influence of indoor factors in dwellings on the development of childhood asthma. *Int. J. Hyg. Environ. Health* **214**, 1–25.

Heran BS, Galm BP, Wright JM (2009) Blood pressure lowering efficacy of alpha blockers for primary hypertension. *Cochrane Database Syst. Rev.* CD004643.

Heran BS, Chen JM, Ebrahim S, Moxham T, Oldridge N, Rees K, Thompson DR, Taylor RS (2011) Exercise-based cardiac rehabilitation for coronary heart disease. *Cochrane Database Syst. Rev.* CD001800.

Himelhoch S, Lehman A, Kreyenbuhl J, Daumit G, Brown C, Dixon L (2004) Prevalence of chronic obstructive pulmonary disease among those with serious mental illness. *Am. J. Psychiatry* **161**, 2317–2319.

Hippisley-Cox J, Pringle M (2005) *Health Inequalities Experienced by People with Schizophrenia and Manic Depression: Analysis of general practice data in England and Wales, Disability Rights Commission.* Available online at: http://disability-studies.leeds.ac.uk/files/library/pringle-Qresearch-initial-analysis-gen-practice-data.pdf (accessed 15 December 2014).

Hodge AM, English DR, O'Dea K, Giles GG (2006) Alcohol intake, consumption pattern and beverage type, and the risk of type 2 diabetes. *Diabet. Med.* **23**, 690–697.

Hofmann SG, Asnaani A, Vonk IJ, Sawyer AT, Fang A (2012) The efficacy of cognitive behavioral therapy: a review of meta-analyses. *Cognit. Ther. Res.* **36**, 427–440.

Howren MB, Lamkin DM, Suls J (2009) Associations of depression with C-reactive protein, IL-1, and IL-6: a meta-analysis. *Psychosom. Med* **71**, 171–186.

Hughes JR (2006) Clinical significance of tobacco withdrawal. *Nicotine Tob. Res.* **8**, 153–156.

Hughes JR (2008) Smoking and suicide: a brief overview. *Drug Alcohol Depend.* **98**, 169–178.

Hughes JR, Stead LF, Hartmann-Boyce J, Cahill K, Lancaster T (2014) Antidepressants for smoking cessation. *Cochrane Database Syst. Rev.* **1**, CD000031.

International Diabetes Institute (2000) *The Asia-Pacific Perspective: Redefining obesity and its treatment.* Caulfield, Victoria, Australia: International Diabetes Institute.

Iqbal N, Lambert T, Masand P (2007) Akathisia: problem of history or concern of today. *CNS Spectr.* **12**, 1–13.

Irving R, Tusie-Luna MT, Mills J, Wright-Pascoe R, McLaughlin W, Aguilar-Salinas CA (2011) Early onset type 2 diabetes in Jamaica and in Mexico. Opportunities derived from an interethnic study. *Rev. Invest. Clin.* **63**, 198–209.

Isbister GK, Buckley NA, Whyte IM (2007) Serotonin toxicity: a practical approach to diagnosis and treatment. *Med. J. Aust.* **187**, 361–365.

Jacka FN, Ystrom E, Brantsaeter AL, Karevold E, Roth C, Haugen M, Meltzer HM, Schjolberg S, Berk M (2013) Maternal and early postnatal nutrition and mental health of offspring by age 5 years: a prospective cohort study. *J. Am. Acad. Child Adolesc. Psychiatry* **52**, 1038–1047.

Jorde R, Sneve M, Figenschau Y, Svartberg J, Waterloo K (2008) Effects of vitamin D supplementation on symptoms of depression in overweight and obese subjects: randomized double blind trial. *J. Intern. Med.* **264**, 599–609.

Julius RJ, Novitsky MA Jr, Dubin WR (2009) Medication adherence: a review of the literature and implications for clinical practice. *J. Psychiatr. Pract.* **15**, 34–44.

Kalra S, Mukherjee JJ, Venkataraman S, Bantwal G, Shaikh S, Saboo B, Das AK, Ramachandran A (2013) Hypoglycemia: the neglected complication. *Ind. J. Endocrinol. Metab.* **17**, 819–834.

Kaludjerovic J, Vieth R (2010) Relationship between vitamin D during perinatal development and health. *J. Midwifery Womens Health* **55**, 550–560.

Kapur S, Remington G (2001) Dopamine D(2) receptors and their role in atypical antipsychotic action: still necessary and may even be sufficient. *Biol. Psychiatry* **50**, 873–883.

Katon WJ (2011) Epidemiology and treatment of depression in patients with chronic medical illness. *Dialogues Clin. Neurosci.* **13**, 7–23.

Kelly GS (2007) Body temperature variability (part 2): masking influences of body temperature variability and a review of body temperature variability in disease. *Altern. Med. Rev.* **12**, 49–62.

Kendler KS, Myers J, Prescott CA (2007) Specificity of genetic and environmental risk factors for symptoms of cannabis, cocaine, alcohol, caffeine, and nicotine dependence. *Arch. Gen. Psychiatry* **64**, 1313–1320.

Kent BD, Grote L, Ryan S, Pepin JL, Bonsignore MR, Tkacova R, Saaresranta T, Verbraecken J, Levy P, Hedner J, McNicholas WT (2014) Diabetes mellitus prevalence and control in sleep disordered breathing: the European Sleep Apnea Cohort (ESADA) study. *Chest* **146**, 982–990.

Kerridge BT, Khan MR, Rehm J, Sapkota A (2014) Terrorism, civil war and related violence and substance use disorder morbidity and mortality: a global analysis. *J. Epidemiol. Glob. Health* **4**, 61–72.

Keshavan MS (1992) Principles of drug therapy in psychiatry: how to do the least harm. In: Keshavan MS, Kennedy JS (eds) *Drug Induced Dysfunction in Psychiatry.* New York: Hemisphere Publishing, pp. 3–8.

Keys A, Fidanza F, Karvonen MJ, Kimura N, Taylor HL (1972) Indices of relative weight and obesity. *J. Chron. Dis.* **25**, 329–343.

Khan LK, Sobush K, Keener D, Goodman K, Lowry A, Kakietek J, Zaro S (2009) Recommended community strategies and measurements to prevent obesity in the United States. *MMWR Recomm. Rep.* **58**, 1–26.

Khandaker GM, Zammit S, Lewis G, Jones PB (2014) A population-based study of atopic disorders and inflammatory markers in childhood before psychotic experiences in adolescence. *Schizophr. Res.* **152**, 139–145.

Khayyam-Nekouei Z, Neshatdoost H, Yousefy A, Sadeghi M, Manshaee G (2013) Psychological factors and coronary heart disease. *ARYA Atheroscler.* **9**, 102–111.

Kim J, Macmaster E, Schwartz TL (2014) Tardive dyskinesia in patients treated with atypical antipsychotics: case series and brief review of etiologic and treatment considerations. *Drugs Context* **2014**, 212259.

Kirsch I, Deacon BJ, Huedo-Medina TB, Scoboria A, Moore TJ, Johnson BT (2008) Initial severity and antidepressant benefits: a meta-analysis of data submitted to the Food and Drug Administration. *PLoS Med.* **5**, e45.

Klein HA, Jackson SM, Street K, Whitacre JC, Klein G (2013) Diabetes self-management education: miles to go 1. *Nurs. Res. Pract.* 581012. Avialable online at: http://www.hindawi.com/journals/nrp/2013/581012 (accessed 15 December 2014).

Komossa K, Rummel-Kluge C, Schwarz S, Schmid F, Hunger H, Kissling W, Leucht S (2011) Risperidone versus other atypical antipsychotics for schizophrenia. *Cochrane Database Syst. Rev.* CD006626.

Kovacs M, Stauder A, Szedmak S (2003) Severity of allergic complaints: the importance of depressed mood. *J. Psychosom. Res.* **54**, 549–557.

Kramer AF, Colcombe SJ, McAuley E, Eriksen KI, Scalf P, Jerome GJ, Marquez DX, Elavsky S, Webb AG (2003) Enhancing brain and cognitive function of older adults through fitness training. *J. Mol. Neurosci.* **20**, 213–221.

Krupnick JL, Sotsky SM, Simmens S, Moyer J, Elkin I, Watkins J, Pilkonis PA (1996) The role of the therapeutic alliance in psychotherapy and pharmacotherapy outcome: findings in the National Institute of Mental Health Treatment of Depression Collaborative Research Program. *J. Consult. Clin. Psychol.* **64**, 532–539.

Krystal AD (2006) Sleep and psychiatric disorders: future directions. *Psychiatr. Clin. North Am.* **29**, 1115–1130.

Kuper H, Marmot M, Hemingway H (2002) Systematic review of prospective cohort studies of psychosocial factors in the etiology and prognosis of coronary heart disease. *Semin. Vasc. Med.* **2**, 267–314.

Kwak SM, Myung SK, Lee YJ, Seo HG (2012) Efficacy of omega-3 fatty acid supplements (eicosapentaenoic acid and docosahexaenoic acid) in the secondary prevention of cardiovascular disease: a meta-analysis of randomized, double-blind, placebo-controlled trials. *Arch. Intern. Med.* **172**, 686–694.

Laamiri FZ, Bouayad A, Otmani A, Ahid S, Mrabet M, Barkat A (2014) Dietery factor obesity microenvironnement and breast cancer. *Gland. Surg.* **3**, 165–173.

Landen M, Hogberg P, Thase ME (2005) Incidence of sexual side effects in refractory depression during treatment with citalopram or paroxetine. *J. Clin. Psychiatry* **66**, 100–106.

Laoutidis ZG, Luckhaus C (2014) 5-HT2A receptor antagonists for the treatment of neuroleptic-induced akathisia: a systematic review and meta-analysis. *Int. J. Neuropsychopharmacol.* **17**, 823–832.

Larson EB, Wang L, Bowen JD, McCormick WC, Teri L, Crane P, Kukull W (2006) Exercise is associated with reduced risk for incident dementia among persons 65 years of age and older. *Ann. Intern. Med.* **144**, 73–81.

Larsson B, Svardsudd K, Welin L, Wilhelmsen L, Bjorntorp P, Tibblin G (1984) Abdominal adipose tissue distribution, obesity, and risk of cardiovascular disease and death: 13 year follow up of participants in the study of men born in 1913. *Br. Med. J. (Clin. Res. Ed.)* **288**, 1401–1404.

Lau RR, Bernard TM, Hartman KA (1989) Further explorations of common-sense representations of common illnesses. *Health Psychol.* **8**, 195–219.

Lavie CJ, Milani RV, Artham SM, Patel DA, Ventura HO (2009) The obesity paradox, weight loss, and coronary disease. *Am. J. Med.* **122**, 1106–1114.

Lawson L, Bridges EJ, Ballou I, Eraker R, Greco S, Shively J, Sochulak V (2007) Accuracy and precision of noninvasive temperature measurement in adult intensive care patients. *Am. J. Crit. Care* **16**, 485–496.

Lee IM (2003) Physical activity and cancer prevention: data from epidemiologic studies. *Med. Sci. Sports Exerc.* **35**, 1823–1827.

Leichsenring F, Salzer S, Jaeger U, Kachele H, Kreische R, Leweke F, Ruger U, Winkelbach C, Leibing E (2009) Short-term psychodynamic psychotherapy and cognitive-behavioral therapy in generalized anxiety disorder: a randomized, controlled trial. *Am. J. Psychiatry* **166**, 875–881.

Lemkes BA, Hermanides J, Devries JH, Holleman F, Meijers JC, Hoekstra JB (2010) Hyperglycemia: a prothrombotic factor? *J. Thromb. Haemost.* **8**, 1663–1669.

Leon DA, McCambridge J (2006) Liver cirrhosis mortality rates in Britain from 1950 to 2002: an analysis of routine data. *Lancet* **367**, 52–56.

Leventhal H, Nerez D, Steele DJ (1984) Illness representations and coping with health threats. In: Baum A, Taylor SE, Singer JE (eds) *Handbook of Psychology and Health: Social psychological aspects of health*. Hillsdale, NJ: Lawrence Erlbaum.

Levy J (1982) A particular kind of negative therapeutic reaction based on Freud's 'borrowed guilt'. *Int. J. Psychoanal.* **63**, 361–368.

Linn MW, Sandifer R, Stein S (1985) Effects of unemployment on mental and physical health. *Am. J. Public Health* **75**, 502–506.

Liu Y, Li Z, Zhang M, Deng Y, Yi Z, Shi T (2013) Exploring the pathogenetic association between schizophrenia and type 2 diabetes mellitus diseases based on pathway analysis. *BMC Med. Genomics* **6** (Suppl 1), S17.

Lopez-Sendon JL, Mena MA, de Yebenes JG (2012) Drug-induced parkinsonism in the elderly: incidence, management and prevention. *Drugs Aging* **29**, 105–118.

Lueboonthavatchai P (2007) Prevalence and psychosocial factors of anxiety and depression in breast cancer patients. *J. Med. Assoc. Thai.* **90**, 2164–2174.

Luengo-Fernandez R, Leal J, Gray A, Petersen S, Rayner M (2006) Cost of cardiovascular diseases in the United Kingdom. *Heart* **92**, 1384–1389.

Luna B, Feinglos MN (2001) Oral agents in the management of type 2 diabetes mellitus. *Am. Fam. Physician* **63**, 1747–1756.

Maddux JE, Rogers RW (1983) Protection motivation theory and self-efficacy: a revised theory of fear appeals and attitude change. *J. Exp. Soc. Psychol.* **19**, 469–479.

Maia AC, Braga AA, Brouwers A, Nardi AE, Oliveira e Silva AC (2012) Prevalence of psychiatric disorders in patients with diabetes types 1 and 2. *Compr. Psychiatry* **53**, 1169–1173.

Mancuso CA, Rincon M, McCulloch CE, Charlson ME (2001) Self-efficacy, depressive symptoms, and patients' expectations predict outcomes in asthma. *Med. Care* **39**, 1326–1338.

Mannino DM, Buist AS (2007) Global burden of COPD: risk factors, prevalence, and future trends. *Lancet* **370**, 765–773.

Marcos A, Manonelles P, Palacios N, Warnberg J, Casajus JA, Perez M, Aznar S, Benito PJ, Martinez-Gomez D, Ortega FB, Ortega E, Urrialde R (2014) Physical activity, hydration and health. *Nutr. Hosp.* **29**, 1224–1239.

Marmot M (2004) The status syndrome. *Significance Statistics Making Sense* **1** (4), 146–192.

Masoro EJ (2005) Overview of caloric restriction and ageing. *Mech. Ageing Dev.* **126**, 913–922.

Mathers CD, Loncar D (2006) Projections of global mortality and burden of disease from 2002 to 2030. *PLoS Med.* **3**, e442.

Matsuoka Y, Nishi D, Yonemoto N, Hamazaki K, Hashimoto K, Hamazaki T (2010) Omega-3 fatty acids for secondary prevention of posttraumatic stress disorder after accidental injury: an open-label pilot study. *J. Clin. Psychopharmacol.* **30**, 217–219.

Mattick RP, Breen C, Kimber J, Davoli M (2009) Methadone maintenance therapy versus no opioid replacement therapy for opioid dependence. *Cochrane Database Syst. Rev.* CD002209.

Mauricio MD, Aldasoro M, Ortega J, Vila JM (2013) Endothelial dysfunction in morbid obesity. *Curr. Pharm. Des.* **19**, 5718–5729.

McCreadie RG (2003) Diet, smoking and cardiovascular risk in people with schizophrenia: descriptive study. *Br. J. Psychiatry* **183**, 534–539.

McNeil C (2001) Cancer advocacy evolves as it gains seats on research panels. *J. Natl Cancer Inst.* **93**, 257–259.

Mechanic D, McAlpine D, Rosenfield S, Davis D (1994) Effects of illness attribution and depression on the quality of life among persons with serious mental illness. *Soc. Sci. Med.* **39**, 155–164.

Meyer JM, Davis VG, Goff DC, McEvoy JP, Nasrallah HA, Davis SM, Rosenheck RA, Daumit GL, Hsiao J, Swartz MS, Stroup TS, Lieberman JA (2008) Change in metabolic syndrome parameters with antipsychotic treatment in the CATIE Schizophrenia Trial: prospective data from phase 1. *Schizophr. Res.* **101**, 273–286.

Mezuk B, Eaton WW, Albrecht S, Golden SH (2008) Depression and type 2 diabetes over the lifespan: a meta-analysis. *Diabetes Care* **31**, 2383–2390.

Miller BJ, Culpepper N, Rapaport MH (2013) C-reactive protein levels in schizophrenia. *Clin. Schizophr. Relat. Psychoses* **7**, 1–22.

Milot J, Meshi B, Taher Shabani RM, Holding G, Mortazavi N, Hayashi S, Hogg JC (2007) The effect of smoking cessation and steroid treatment on emphysema in guinea pigs. *Respir. Med.* **101**, 2327–2335.

Minozzi S, Davoli M, Bargagli AM, Amato L, Vecchi S, Perucci CA (2010) An overview of systematic reviews on cannabis and psychosis: discussing apparently conflicting results. *Drug Alcohol Rev.* **29**, 304–317.

Mishra SI, Scherer RW, Geigle PM, Berlanstein DR, Topaloglu O, Gotay CC, Snyder C (2012) Exercise interventions on health-related quality of life for cancer survivors. *Cochrane Database Syst. Rev.* **8**, CD007566.

Mlyniec K, Budziszewska B, Reczynski W, Doboszewska U, Pilc A, Nowak G (2013) Zinc deficiency alters responsiveness to antidepressant drugs in mice. *Pharmacol. Rep.* **65**, 579–592.

Moore PE, Ryckman KK, Williams SM, Patel N, Summar ML, Sheller JR (2009) Genetic variants of GSNOR and ADRB2 influence response to albuterol in African-American children with severe asthma. *Pediatr. Pulmonol.* **44**, 649–654.

Morkedal B, Romundstad PR, Vatten LJ (2011) Mortality from ischaemic heart disease: age-specific effects of blood pressure stratified by body-mass index: the HUNT cohort study in Norway. *J. Epidemiol. Commun. Hlth* **65**, 814–819.

Mrazek DA (1992) Psychiatric complications of pediatric asthma. *Ann. Allergy* **69**, 285–290.

Mukai T, Kishi T, Matsuda Y, Iwata N (2014) A meta-analysis of inositol for depression and anxiety disorders. *Hum. Psychopharmacol.* **29**, 55–63.

Muller N (2014) Immunology of major depression. *Neuroimmunomodulation* **21**, 123–130.

Munoz MA, Fito M, Marrugat J, Covas MI, Schroder H (2009) Adherence to the Mediterranean diet is associated with better mental and physical health. *Br. J. Nutr.* **101**, 1821–1827.

Munro I, Edward KL (2008) Mental illness and substance use: an Australian perspective. *Int. J. Ment. Health Nurs.* **17**, 255–260.

Mutsatsa S (2011) *Medicines Management in Mental Health Nursing: Transforming practice.* Exeter: Learning Matters.

Nanri A, Mizoue T, Poudel-Tandukar K, Noda M, Kato M, Kurotani K, Goto A, Oba S, Inoue M, Tsugane S (2013) Dietary patterns and suicide in Japanese adults: the Japan Public Health Center-based prospective study. *Br. J. Psychiatry* **203**, 422–427.

Naranjo CA, Busto U, Sellers EM, Sandor P, Ruiz I, Roberts EA, Janecek E, Domecq C, Greenblatt DJ (1981) A method for estimating the probability of adverse drug reactions. *Clin. Pharmacol. Ther.* **30**, 239–245.

Nasrallah HA, Meyer JM, Goff DC, McEvoy JP, Davis SM, Stroup TS, Lieberman JA (2006a) Low rates of treatment for hypertension, dyslipidemia and diabetes in schizophrenia: data from the CATIE schizophrenia trial sample at baseline. *Schizophr. Res.* **86**, 15–22.

Nasrallah HA, Meyer JM, Goff DC, McEvoy JP, Davis SM, Stroup TS, Lieberman JA (2006b) Low rates of treatment for hypertension, dyslipidemia and diabetes in schizophrenia: data from the CATIE schizophrenia trial sample at baseline. *Schizophr. Res.* **86**, 15–22.

National Clinical Guidelines Centre (2010) *Alcohol Use Disorders: Diagnosis and clinical management of alcohol-related physical complications.* London: The Royal College of Physicians.

Nazare JA, Smith JD, Borel AL, Haffner SM, Balkau B, Ross R, Massien C, Almeras N, Despres JP (2012) Ethnic influences on the relations between abdominal subcutaneous and visceral adiposity, liver fat, and cardiometabolic risk profile: the International Study of Prediction of Intra-Abdominal Adiposity and its Relationship with Cardiometabolic Risk/Intra-Abdominal Adiposity. *Am. J. Clin. Nutr.* **96**, 714–726.

Newcomer JW (2005) Second-generation (atypical) antipsychotics and metabolic effects: a comprehensive literature review. *CNS Drugs* **19** (Suppl 1), 1–93.

NHS Choices (2013) *Physical Activity Guidelines for Adults.* Available online at: http://www.nhs.uk/Livewell/fitness/Pages/physical-activity-guidelines-for-adults.aspx (accessed 15 December 2014).

NICE (2007a) *MI – Secondary Prevention: Secondary prevention in primary and secondary care for patients following a myocardial infarction.* Available online at: http://www.nice.org.uk/guidance/cg48 (accessed 9 December 2014).

NICE (2007b) *Methadone and Buprenorphine for the Management of Opioid Dependence.* Available online at: http://www.nice.org.uk/guidance/ta114 (accessed 15 December 2014).

NICE (2008) *Public Health Guidance: Reducing the rate of premature deaths from cardiovascular disease and other smoking related diseases: Finding and supporting those most at risk and improving access to services.* Available online at: http://www.nice.org.uk/guidance/ph15/resources/guidance-identifying-and-supporting-people-most-at-risk-of-dying-prematurely-pdf (accessed 15 December 2014).

NICE (2009a) *The NICE Guidelines on the Treatment and Management of Depression* (updated edition). London: National Health Service.

NICE (2009b) *Type 2 Diabetes: The management of type 2 diabetes.* London: National Institute for Health and Care Excellence.

NMC (2010) *Standards for Pre-registration Nursing.* London: Nursing and Midwifery Council.

Nocon A, Rhodes PJ, Wright JP, Eastham J, Williams DR, Harrison SR, Young RJ (2004) Specialist general practitioners and diabetes clinics in primary care: a qualitative and descriptive evaluation. *Diabet. Med.* **21**, 32–38.

Nutt D (1999) Alcohol and the brain. Pharmacological insights for psychiatrists. *Br. J. Psychiatry* **175**, 114–119.

O'Donnell M, Teo K, Gao P, Anderson C, Sleight P, Dans A, Marzona I, Bosch J, Probstfield J, Yusuf S (2012) Cognitive impairment and risk of cardiovascular events and mortality. *Eur. Heart J.* **33**, 1777–1786.

Ohman H, Savikko N, Strandberg TE, Pitkala KH (2014) Effect of physical exercise on cognitive performance in older adults with mild cognitive impairment or dementia: a systematic review. *Dement. Geriatr. Cogn. Disord.* **38**, 347–365.

Orozco LJ, Buchleitner AM, Gimenez-Perez G, Roque IF, Richter B, Mauricio D (2008) Exercise or exercise and diet for preventing type 2 diabetes mellitus. *Cochrane Database Syst. Rev.* CD003054.

Oyesanmi O, Snyder D, Sullivan N, Reston J, Treadwell J, Schoelles KM (2010) Alcohol consumption and cancer risk: understanding possible causal mechanisms for breast and colorectal cancers. *Evid. Rep. Technol. Assess. (Full Rep.)*, 1–151.

Palmefors H, DuttaRoy S, Rundqvist B, Borjesson M (2014) The effect of physical activity or exercise on key biomarkers in atherosclerosis: a systematic review. *Atherosclerosis* **235**, 150–161.

Pan A, Sun Q, Okereke OI, Rexrode KM, Hu FB (2011) Depression and risk of stroke morbidity and mortality: a meta-analysis and systematic review. *J.A.M.A.* **306**, 1241–1249.

Papanastasiou E (2012) Interventions for the metabolic syndrome in schizophrenia: a review. *Ther. Adv. Endocrinol. Metab* **3**, 141–162.

Parasuramalu BG, Huliraj N, Prashanth Kumar SP, Ramesh Masthi NR, Srinivasa Babu CR (2014) Prevalence of chronic obstructive pulmonary disease and its association with tobacco smoking and environmental tobacco smoke exposure among rural population. *Ind. J. Public Health* **58**, 45–49.

Pasco JA, Jacka FN, Williams LJ, Evans-Cleverdon M, Brennan SL, Kotowicz MA, Nicholson GC, Ball MJ, Berk M (2012) Dietary selenium and major depression: a nested case-control study. *Complement Ther. Med.* **20**, 119–123.

Pearce SH, Cheetham TD (2010) Diagnosis and management of vitamin D deficiency. *BMJ* **340**, b5664.

Pedersen MS, Benros ME, Agerbo E, Borglum AD, Mortensen PB (2012) Schizophrenia in patients with atopic disorders with particular emphasis on asthma: a Danish population-based study. *Schizophr. Res.* **138**, 58–62.

Peet M (2004) International variations in the outcome of schizophrenia and the prevalence of depression in relation to national dietary practices: an ecological analysis. *Br. J. Psychiatry* **184**, 404–408.

Pham NM, Nanri A, Kurotani K, Kuwahara K, Kume A, Sato M, Hayabuchi H, Mizoue T (2014) Green tea and coffee consumption is inversely associated with depressive symptoms in a Japanese working population. *Public Health Nutr.* **17**, 625–633.

Phelan M, Stradins L, Morrison S (2001) Physical health of people with severe mental illness. *BMJ* **322**, 443–444.

Phillips GT, Gossop M, Bradley B (1986) The influence of psychological factors on the opiate withdrawal syndrome. *Br. J. Psychiatry* **149**, 235–238.

Pilote L, Tu JV, Humphries K, Behouli H, Belisle P, Austin PC, Joseph L (2007) Socioeconomic status, access to health care, and outcomes after acute myocardial infarction in Canada's universal health care system. *Med. Care* **45**, 638–646.

Pimenta F, Leal I, Maroco J, Ramos C (2012) Brief cognitive-behavioral therapy for weight loss in midlife women: a controlled study with follow-up 5. *Int. J. Womens Health* **4**, 559–567.

Potoczek A, Nizankowska-Mogilnicka E, Bochenek G, Szczeklik A (2006) Difficult asthma and gender of patients versus the presence of profound psychological trauma. *Psychiatr. Pol.* **40**, 1081–1096.

Poyurovsky M (2010) Acute antipsychotic-induced akathisia revisited. *Br. J. Psychiatry* **196**, 89–91.

Prasad AS (2014) Zinc: an antioxidant and anti-inflammatory agent: role of zinc in degenerative disorders of aging. *J. Trace Elem. Med. Biol.* **28**, 364–371.

Pretty J, Peacock J, Sellens M, Griffin M (2005) The mental and physical health outcomes of green exercise. *Int. J. Environ. Health Res.* **15**, 319–337.

Prochaska JO, DiClemente CC (1984) Self change processes, self efficacy and decisional balance across five stages of smoking cessation. *Prog. Clin. Biol. Res.* **156**, 131–140.

Rana AQ, Chaudry ZM, Blanchet PJ (2013) New and emerging treatments for symptomatic tardive dyskinesia. *Drug Des. Devel. Ther.* **7**, 1329–1340.

Rank MA, Hagan JB, Park MA, Podjasek JC, Samant SA, Volcheck GW, Erwin PJ, West CP (2013) The risk of asthma exacerbation after stopping low-dose inhaled corticosteroids: a systematic review and meta-analysis of randomized controlled trials. *J. Allergy Clin. Immunol.* **131**, 724–729.

Reynolds M, Mezey G, Chapman M, Wheeler M, Drummond C, Baldacchino A (2005) Co-morbid post-traumatic stress disorder in a substance misusing clinical population. *Drug Alcohol Depend.* **77**, 251–258.

Rice VH, Stead LF (2008) Nursing interventions for smoking cessation. *Cochrane Database Syst. Rev.* CD001188.

Rinomhota AS, Cooper K (1996) Homeostasis: restoring the internal wellbeing in patients/clients. *Br. J. Nurs.* **5**, 1100–1108.

Ryan MC, Thakore JH (2002) Physical consequences of schizophrenia and its treatment: the metabolic syndrome. *Life Sci.* **71**, 239–257.

Sachdev P (1995) The development of the concept of akathisia: a historical overview. *Schizophr. Res.* **16**, 33–45.

Safran JD, Segal ZV (1996) *Interpersonal Process in Cognitive Therapy.* Oxford: Rowman & Littelfields.

Sampson EL, Gould V, Lee D, Blanchard MR (2006) Differences in care received by patients with and without dementia who died during acute hospital admission: a retrospective case note study. *Age Ageing* **35**, 187–189.

Sanchez-Villegas A, Doreste J, Schlatter J, Pla J, Bes-Rastrollo M, Martinez-Gonzalez MA (2009) Association between folate, vitamin B(6) and vitamin B(12) intake and depression in the SUN cohort study. *J. Hum. Nutr. Diet* **22**, 122–133.

Schatzberg AF, Haddad P, Kaplan EM, Lejoyeux M, Rosenbaum JF, Young AH, Zajecka J (1997) Serotonin reuptake inhibitor discontinuation syndrome: a hypothetical definition. Discontinuation Consensus panel. *J. Clin. Psychiatry* **58** (Suppl 7), 5–10.

Schoepf D, Potluri R, Uppal H, Natalwala A, Narendran P, Heun R (2012) Type-2 diabetes mellitus in schizophrenia: increased prevalence and major risk factor of excess mortality in a naturalistic 7-year follow-up. *Eur. Psychiatry* **27**, 33–42.

Schoepf D, Uppal H, Potluri R, Heun R (2014) Physical comorbidity and its relevance on mortality in schizophrenia: a naturalistic 12-year follow-up in general hospital admissions. *Eur. Arch. Psychiatry Clin. Neurosci.* **264**, 3–28.

Schonecker M (1957) Paroxysmal dyskinesia as the effect of megaphen. *Nervenarzt* **28** (12), 550–553.

Schuckit MA, Tipp JE, Reich T, Hesselbrock VM, Bucholz KK (1995) The histories of withdrawal convulsions and delirium tremens in 1648 alcohol dependent subjects. *Addiction* **90**, 1335–1347.

Seeman M, Seeman TE (1983) Health behavior and personal autonomy: a longitudinal study of the sense of control in illness. *J. Health Soc. Behav.* **24**, 144–160.

Seguin B, Hardy B, Singer PA, Daar AS (2008) Bidil: recontextualizing the race debate. *Pharmacogenomics J.* **8**, 169–173.

Shabbir F, Patel A, Mattison C, Bose S, Krishnamohan R, Sweeney E, Sandhu S, Nel W, Rais A, Sandhu R, Ngu N, Sharma S (2013) Effect of diet on serotonergic neurotransmission in depression. *Neurochem. Int.* **62**, 324–329.

Shen MM, Abate-Shen C (2010) Molecular genetics of prostate cancer: new prospects for old challenges. *Genes Dev.* **24**, 1967–2000.

Shephard RJ, Futcher R (1997) Physical activity and cancer: how may protection be maximized? *Crit. Rev. Oncog.* **8**, 219–272.

Shirani F, Salehi-Abargouei A, Azadbakht L (2013) Effects of Dietary Approaches to Stop Hypertension (DASH) diet on some risk for developing type 2 diabetes: a systematic review and meta-analysis on controlled clinical trials. *Nutrition* **29**, 939–947.

Simpson KA, Singh MA (2008) Effects of exercise on adiponectin: a systematic review. *Obesity (Silver Spring)* **16**, 241–256.

Sloboda Z, Glantz MD, Tarter RE (2012) Revisiting the concepts of risk and protective factors for understanding the etiology and development of substance use and substance use disorders: implications for prevention. *Subst. Use Misuse* **47**, 944–962.

Smith PH, Mazure CM, McKee SA (2014) Smoking and mental illness in the US population. *Tob. Control* **23**, e147–e153.

Sofi F, Macchi C, Abbate R, Gensini GF, Casini A (2013) Mediterranean diet and health status: an updated meta-analysis and a proposal for a literature-based adherence score. *Public Health Nutr.* 1–14.

Solati Z, Jazayeri S, Tehrani-Doost M, Mahmoodianfard S, Gohari MR (2014) Zinc monotherapy increases serum brain-derived neurotrophic factor (BDNF) levels and decreases depressive symptoms in overweight or obese subjects: A double-blind, randomized, placebo-controlled trial. *Nutr. Neurosci.* (epub ahead of print).

Solfrizzi V, Panza F (2014) Mediterranean diet and cognitive decline. A lesson from the whole-diet approach: what challenges lie ahead? *J. Alzheimers Dis.* **39**, 283–286.

Stahl S (2008) *Stahl's Essential Psychopharmacology: Neuroscientific basis and practical application.* Cambridge: Cambridge University Press.

Stanley S, Laugharne J (2014) The impact of lifestyle factors on the physical health of people with a mental illness: a brief review. *Int. J. Behav. Med.* **21**, 275–281.

Stead LF, Perera R, Lancaster T (2007) A systematic review of interventions for smokers who contact quit-lines. *Tob. Control* **16** (Suppl 1), i3–i8.

Stead LF, Perera R, Bullen C, Mant D, Hartmann-Boyce J, Cahill K, Lancaster T (2012) Nicotine replacement therapy for smoking cessation. *Cochrane Database Syst. Rev.* **11**, CD000146.

Stephens JH, Ota KY, Carpenter WT, Jr, Shaffer JW (1980) Diagnostic criteria for schizophrenia: prognostic implications and diagnostic overlap. *Psychiatry Res.* **2**, 1–12.

Strachan DP (2000) Family size, infection and atopy: the first decade of the 'hygiene hypothesis'. *Thorax* **55** (Suppl 1), S2–10.

Strachan JG, Stuckey NA (1989) Early experience in the establishment of an integrated psychiatric day hospital. *Health Bull. (Edinb.)* **47**, 133–140.

Strang J, Marks I, Dawe S, Powell J, Gossop M, Richards D, Gray J (1997) Type of hospital setting and treatment outcome with heroin addicts. Results from a randomised trial. *Br. J. Psychiatry* **171**, 335–339.

Strasser AA, Kaufmann V, Jepson C, Perkins KA, Pickworth WB, Wileyto EP, Rukstalis M, Audrain-McGovern J, Lerman C (2005) Effects of different nicotine replacement therapies on postcessation psychological responses. *Addict. Behav.* **30**, 9–17.

Stroke Association (2006) *What is a Stroke?* Available online at: http://mhfs.org.uk/resources/NMHW06/pdf/What_is_a_stroke.pdf (accessed 15 December 2014).

Sturdy PM, Victor CR, Anderson HR, Bland JM, Butland BK, Harrison BD, Peckitt C, Taylor JC (2002) Psychological, social and health behaviour risk factors for deaths certified as asthma: a national case-control study. *Thorax* **57**, 1034–1039.

Swanson KM (1991) Empirical development of a middle range theory of caring. *Nursing Res.* **40** (3), 161–166.

Taras H, Potts-Datema W (2005) Sleep and student performance at school. *J. Sch. Health* **75**, 248–254.

Taylor D, Paton C, Kerwin R (2007). Substance misuse. In: Taylor D, Paton C, Kerwin R (eds) *Maudsley Prescribing Guidelines*, 9th edn. London: Informa Healthcare, pp. 302–352.

Taylor JY, Wu CY, Darling D, Sun YV, Kardia SL, Jackson JS (2012) Gene–environment effects of SLC4A5 and skin color on blood pressure among African American women. *Ethn. Dis.* **22**, 155–161.

The Health and Social Care Information Centre (2012) *Statistics on Smoking: England.* Available online at: http://www.hscic.gov.uk/catalogue/PUB14988/smok-eng-2014-rep.pdf (accessed 15 December 2014).

Thompson CJ, Boddy K, Stein K, Whear R, Barton J, Depledge MH (2011) Does participating in physical activity in outdoor natural environments have a greater effect on physical and mental wellbeing than physical activity indoors? A systematic review. *Environ. Sci. Technol.* **45**, 1761–1772.

Tordeurs D, Janne P, Appart A, Zdanowicz N, Reynaert C (2011) Effectiveness of physical exercise in psychiatry: a therapeutic approach? *Encephale* **37**, 345–352.

Toth PP (2005) Cardiology patient page. The 'good cholesterol': high-density lipoprotein. *Circulation* **111**, e89–e91.

Trifiro G (2011) Antipsychotic drug use and community-acquired pneumonia. *Curr. Infect. Dis. Rep.* **13**, 262–268.

Tsai KY, Lee CC, Chou YM, Su CY, Chou FH (2012) The incidence and relative risk of stroke in patients with schizophrenia: a five-year follow-up study. *Schizophr. Res.* **138**, 41–47.

Turner JB (1995) Economic context and the health effect of unemployed. *J. Hlth Social Beha.* **36**, 213–229.

Umpierre D, Ribeiro PA, Kramer CK, Leitao CB, Zucatti AT, Azevedo MJ, Gross JL, Ribeiro JP, Schaan BD (2011) Physical activity advice only or structured exercise training and association with HbA1c levels in type 2 diabetes: a systematic review and meta-analysis. *J.A.M.A.* **305**, 1790–1799.

US Department of Health and Human Services (2004) *The Health Consequences of Smoking: A report of the Surgeon General.* Atlanta: US Department of Health and Human Services, Centers for Disease Control and Prevention, National Center for Chronic Disease Prevention and Health Promotion, Office on Smoking and Health.

Vivekananthan DP, Penn MS, Sapp SK, Hsu A, Topol EJ (2003) Use of antioxidant vitamins for the prevention of cardiovascular disease: meta-analysis of randomised trials. *Lancet* **361**, 2017–2023.

Volaklis KA, Halle M, Tokmakidis SP (2013) Exercise in the prevention and rehabilitation of breast cancer. *Wien. Klin. Wochenschr.* **125**, 297–301.

Volkov VP (2009) Respiratory diseases as a cause of death in schizophrenia. *Probl. Tuberk. Bolezn. Legk.* 24–27.

Wamboldt MZ, Weintraub P, Krafchick D, Wamboldt FS (1996) Psychiatric family history in adolescents with severe asthma. *J. Am. Acad. Child Adolesc. Psychiatry* **35**, 1042–1049.

Watanabe Y, Someya T, Nawa H (2010) Cytokine hypothesis of schizophrenia pathogenesis: evidence from human studies and animal models. *Psychiatry Clin. Neurosci.* **64**, 217–230.

Watkins LL, Koch GG, Sherwood A, Blumenthal JA, Davidson JR, O'Connor C, Sketch MH (2013) Association of anxiety and depression with all-cause mortality in individuals with coronary heart disease. *J. Am. Heart Assoc.* **2**, e000068.

Weber NS, Cowan DN, Millikan AM, Niebuhr DW (2009) Psychiatric and general medical conditions comorbid with schizophrenia in the National Hospital Discharge Survey. *Psychiatr. Serv.* **60**, 1059–1067.

Weissman MM, Warner V, Wickramaratne PJ, Kandel DB (1999) Maternal smoking during pregnancy and psychopathology in offspring followed to adulthood. *J. Am. Acad. Child Adolesc. Psychiatry* **38**, 892–899.

West R, Shiffman S (2001) Effect of oral nicotine dosing forms on cigarette withdrawal symptoms and craving: a systematic review. *Psychopharmacology (Berl)* **155**, 115–122.

White HD, Aylward PE, Frey MJ, Adgey AA, Nair R, Hillis WS, Shalev Y, Brown MA, French JK, Collins R, Maraganore J, Adelman B (1997) Randomized, double-blind comparison of hirulog versus heparin in patients receiving streptokinase and aspirin for acute myocardial infarction (HERO). Hirulog Early Reperfusion/Occlusion (HERO) trial investigators. *Circulation* **96**, 2155–2161.

WHO (1992) *The ICD–10 Classification of Mental and Behavioural Disorders: Clinical Descriptions and Diagnostic Guidelines.* Geneva: World Health Organization.

WHO (1995) *Physical Status: The use and interpretation of apometry.* Geneva: WHO.

WHO (2003a) *Prevention of Allergy and Allergic Asthma.* Geneva: World Health Organization.

WHO (2003b) *Global Cancer Rates Could Increase by 50% to 15 Million by 2020.* Geneva: World Health Organization.

WHO (2005) *Tobacco Free Initiative Report.* Geneva: World Health Organization.

WHO (2008a) *Primary Health Care: Now more than ever.* Geneva: World Health Organization.

WHO (2008b) *Waist Circumference and Waist–Hip Ratio: Report of a WHO expert consultation.* Geneva: WHO.

WHO (2009) *Milestones in Health Promotion: Statements from global conferences.* Geneva: Word Health Organization Press.

WHO (2011a) *Global Status Report on Noncommunicable Disease.* Geneva: World Health Organization.

WHO (2011b) *World Health Statistics 2008.* Geneva: World Health Organization.

WHO (2011c) *Global Atlas on Cardiovascular Disease Prevention and Control.* Geneva: World Health Organization.

WHO (2011d) *Global Status Report on Alcohol and Health.* Geneva: World Health Organization.

WHO (2014a) *Health Promotion.* Available online at: http://www.who.int/healthpromotion/en (accessed 15 December 2014).

WHO (2014b) *Management of Substance Abuse: Facts and figures.* Geneva: World Health Organization.

WHO (2014c) *Stroke, Cerebrovascular Accident.* Geneva: World Health Organization.

Wiehl WO, Hayner G, Galloway G (1994) Haight Ashbury Free Clinics' drug detoxification protocols – Part 4: Alcohol. *J. Psychoactive Drugs* **26**, 57–59.

Wilkinson RG, Marmot MG (2003) *Social Determinants of Health: The solid facts.* Copenhagen: World Health Organization.

Willcox DC, Scapagnini G, Willcox BJ (2014) Healthy aging diets other than the Mediterranean: a focus on the Okinawan diet. *Mech. Ageing Dev.* **136–137**, 148–162.

References

Willcox DC, Willcox BJ, Todoriki H, Suzuki M (2009) The Okinawan diet: health implications of a low-calorie, nutrient-dense, antioxidant-rich dietary pattern low in glycemic load. *J. Am. Coll. Nutr.* **28** (Suppl), 500S–516S.

Williams JM, Foulds J (2007) Successful tobacco dependence treatment in schizophrenia. *Am. J. Psychiatry* **164**, 222–227.

Willis T (1971) *Diabetes: A medical odyssey.* New York: Tuckahoe.

Wiltink J, Dippel A, Szczepanski M, Thiede R, Alt C, Beutel ME (2007) Long-term weight loss maintenance after inpatient psychotherapy of severely obese patients based on a randomized study: predictors and maintaining factors of health behavior. *J. Psychosom. Res.* **62**, 691–698.

Woerner MG, Alvir JM, Saltz BL, Lieberman JA, Kane JM (1998) Prospective study of tardive dyskinesia in the elderly: rates and risk factors. *Am. J. Psychiatry* **155**, 1521–1528.

World Health Organization (1998) *List of Basic Terms.* Available online at: http://www.who.int/healthpromotion/about/HPR%20Glossary%201998.pdf (accessed 15 December 2014).

World Health Organization (2004) *BMI Classification.* Available online at: http://apps.who.int/bmi/index.jsp?introPage=intro_3.html (accessed 15 December 2014).

Yogaratnam J, Biswas N, Vadivel R, Jacob R (2013) Metabolic complications of schizophrenia and antipsychotic medications – an updated review. *East Asian Arch. Psychiatry* **23**, 21–28.

Zomer E, Owen A, Magliano DJ, Liew D, Reid C (2011) Validation of two Framingham cardiovascular risk prediction algorithms in an Australian population: the 'old' versus the 'new' Framingham equation. *Eur. J. Cardiovasc. Prev. Rehabil.* **18**, 115–120.

Index